The Best of
Health
Professions
Humor

Jean Scholz

The Best of Health Professions Humor

A Collection of Articles, Essays, and Poetry Published in the Allied Health Literature

COMPILED AND EDITED BY
COLLEEN KENEFICK

ASSOCIATE LIBRARIAN, HEALTH SCIENCES CENTER LIBRARY
STATE UNIVERSITY OF NEW YORK AT STONY BROOK
STONY BROOK, NEW YORK

HANLEY & BELFUS, INC.
PHILADELPHIA

Publisher: HANLEY & BELFUS, INC.
               Medical Publishers
               210 South 13th Street
               Philadelphia, PA 19107
               (215) 546-7293; 800-962-1892
               FAX (215) 790-9330
               Web site: http://www.hanleyandbelfus.com

Library of Congress Cataloging-in-Publication Data

The best of health professions humor : a collection of articles, essays, and poetry published in the allied health literature / compiled and edited by Colleen Kenefick.
    p. ; cm.
Includes index.
ISBN 1-56053-457-5 (alk. paper)
   1. Medicine—Humor.   I. Kenefick, Colleen.
[DNLM: 1. Allied Health Occupations—Collected Works.   2. Allied Health Occupations—Humor.   WZ 305 B56125 2001]
R705.B43 2001
610'.2'07—dc21

00-058092

The Best of Health Professions Humor   ISBN 1-56053-457-5

© 2001 by Hanley & Belfus, Inc. All rights reserved. No part of this book may be reproduced, reused, re-published, or transmitted in any form or by any means without written permission of the publisher.

Last digit is the print number: 9 8 7 6 5 4 3 2 1

DEDICATION

To my husband, Erwin London,
who continues to be
my first and best reader.

CONTENTS

Acknowledgments   xiii

Introduction   xv

IT'S NEWS TO ME

The News from Lake Mindbegone . . . 3
J. RUSSELL TEAGARDEN, MA

Tabloid Medicine and the
Medical Options Market . . . 5
DAVID WOLMAN, PA-C

Instructions for Editors:
A "Revenge Fantasy" . . . 7
JOSEPH HERMAN

How to Kill an Association . . . 8
ANONYMOUS

A Different Kind of Turf Battle . . . 9
JULES M. ROTHSTEIN, PhD, PT

Try Ignorance . . . 10
GABOR B. LEVY

That's Entertainment . . . 11
NEAL A. WHITMAN, EdD

Danger in the Newsroom . . . 13
KEVIN SHEA O'MALLEY, RPh

Nietzsche and the Evening News . . . 15
STEVEN TIGER, PA

Letter from America: Quis
Custodiet Ipsos Custodes? . . . 17
STUART A. BENTLEY

So You've Joined A Society . . . 18
ANONYMOUS

Dear Mr. Brown . . . 19
RUSSELL L. MALONE

Pharmacy's New (Starring) Role . . . 21
DOUG BENNETT, RPh

TODAY MIGHT BE DIFFERENT

You Say You Want a Resolution? . . . 25
JEFF LUCIA, NREMT-P

Be a Lean, Mean, Filling Machine . . . 26
DOUG BENNETT, RPh

Summer Advice: More
Than Just Sunscreen . . . 27
MONTGOMERY VICKERS, OD

Hello Mudda, Hello Fadda . . .
A Letter from Camp PT . . . 29
PETER KOVACEK, MS, PT

Camp PT Is Looking Better . . . 30
DAN DANDY, PT

An Ode to Call Technologists . . . 31
ANONYMOUS

Bathroom Humor . . . 32
KATHY SITZMAN, BSN, RN

Your Guide to Feigning Civility . . . 33
BARBARA M. MORRIS, RPh

A Is for Aardvark . . . 34
DANIEL MERTON

Fast! Warm! Fuzzy! Emergency! . . . 35
DAVID WOLMAN, PA-C

Laws of the O.R. . . . 39
MARCH L. WARN, RN, CNOR

The Zen of Pharmacy . . . 40
JIM PLAGAKIS, RPh

Stop Working So Hard.
Get Yourself Fired . . . 41
CAMPION QUINN, MD

SPEAKING PATIENTLY

Gone Fishing . . . 45
JEANNETTE WOLFE, MD

Sizzling Secret Clinical Confessions . . . 46
STEVEN TIGER, PA

Pre-Op Instructions as
Our Patients Hear Them . . . 47
MARCH L. WARN, RN

My Dog Ate My Running Shoes:
Fitness Excuses from Patients . . . 49
AMBER STENGER

Not Just Window Dressing:
Gowns as the Latest Fashion . . . 50
PAM JOHNSON, BS, RT(R)

Unrecalled Falls . . . 51
JEFF BRONE

Finding Humor in Our Workplace . . . 52
SHARON P. HALL, RNC

Mandatory Infection
Out-of-Control Test . . . 53
STEVEN J. SCHWEON
EILEEN O'ROURKE
SUSAN TROUT
ROBERT QUINN-O'CONNOR
ELAINE NEELY

Just a Number, Or Is It? . . . 55
CLIFF THOMAS, RPh

The Drag and Nag Method
of Gait Training . . . 56
MARTHA SOMERS, PT

Bugs Are Not Funny Syndrome . . . 57
STEVEN J. SCHWEON, RN, MPH
ELLEN NOVATNACK, RN, BSN
EILEEN O'ROURKE, MT(ASCP), CIC
SUSAN TROUT, RN, CIC

TRADING PLACES

How to Visit the Doctor . . . 61
HOWARD J. BENNETT, MD

The 12 Puffs of Christmas . . . 62
WARREN MCNAB

Learning to Wait with Dignity . . . 63
VALENTINE CARDINALE

An ER Patient's Complaint . . . 64
B. VÖN KOLN KLEINMÜNTZ

Syphilis . . . 65
VICTOR F. TAPSON

What to Do When You're Sick . . . 66
BILL OTT

Confessions of a Street Medic . . . 67
JEFF MCBRAYER

Oncologists and Radiologists . . . 69
ARTHUR W. DEVERMANN

MANAGING TO CARE

First, Do No Harm
(Pending Prior Approval) . . . 73
ALEC PRUCHNICKI, MD

Breast Reduction Ad Absurdum . . . 75
ROBERT M. GOLDWYN, MD

Up to Your Waist in Alligators? . . . 77
BARBARA PENN, BSc, DipCOT, SROT, CMS

Pharmacy-Buzzword Bingo . . . 78
BRUCE A. MUELLER, PharmD, FCCP
BRUCE C. CARLSTEDT, PhD

A Modest Proposal: A Satirical
Look at Managed Care . . . 79
JAMES F. LALLY, MD

I've Become the Perfect HMO Provider! . . . 80
STANLEY J. SAVINESE, DO

A Pop Quiz . . . 82
MARY GRAYSON

Adventures in the PA Trade . . . 83
DAVID WOLMAN, PA-C

A Healthcare Parable . . . 85
WILLIAM R. PENTECOST, NREMT-P

In the Push to Explore New Frontiers . . . 86
LYNN WAGNER

The MacPherson
Triangulation Technique . . . 87
LEO A. GORDON, MD, FACS

A Clinic for Everyone . . . 89
ROBERT M. GOLDWYN, MD

Hal Revisited . . . 90
MARY GRAYSON

WHAT IT REALLY MEANS

Can We Talk? . . . 93
ELIZABETH A. J. HASEGAWA, PharmD

Effect on Human Longevity
of Added Dietary Chocolate . . . 94
JOEL KIRSCHBAUM, PhD

Words that Deny Reality . . . 95
JULES M. ROTHSTEIN, PhD, PT, FAPTA

Tips for Interpreting "Science-Speak" . . . 97
ANONYMOUS

Bits, Bytes, and Middle Age . . . 98
VICTOR INCE, ART

Media Lament . . . 99
KAREN H. MORIN, DSN, RN

On the Other Side of the
Research Looking Glass . . . 100
MARK RADCLIFFE

The Beeper, and Its Use
in Mating Displays . . . 101
BRUCE CARLSON

Sleep Research Update . . . 102
YUSKA-MARIE PASKEVITCH

Don't Put Your Footnotes
in Your Mouth . . . 103
DAVID WOLMAN, PA-C

The Ugly Side of Peer Review . . . 105
JULES M. ROTHSTEIN, PhD, PT, FAPTA

Nickels and Dimes . . . 107
LEONARD LASTER

Information Management Truths
in Small Bytes . . . 109
BRUCE A. FRIEDMAN, MD

CHAINS OF COMMAND

Interviewers Are "Like a Box of Chocolates":
You Never Know Who You'll Get . . . 113
THOMAS W. O'CONNOR, PharmD, MBA

The Day Hell Froze Over
in the Medical Laboratory . . . 114
MICHAEL RAMSEY, PhD, MT(ASCP), CLS(NCA)

Team Building . . . 115
STEVE NOWAK, RT(R), MBA

How to Read a Collective Bargaining
Contract: The Lighter Side of
the Management View . . . 117
JOAN GEETTER

The Importance of Being
Like Ernest . . . 119
SANJIVA WIJESINHA

A Chilling Tale . . . 120
SIRENHEAD

Reengineering for the Birds . . . 121
DARLENE SREDL

The Indestructible
Bacillus Bureaucraticus . . . 123
ROBERT M. GOLDWYN, MD

The Organization Zoo: A Fable . . . 125
JOHN G. BRUHN, PhD
ALAN P. CHESNEY, PhD

How to Enjoy Being a Chair . . . 127
ANNE PARRY, PhD, MCSP, DipTP

What's in a Name? . . . 128
MICHAEL J. SHAFFER, DSc

THE MORE THINGS CHANGE

Message to a Graduating Class
and None Should Fail . . . 131
H. F. Helmholz Jr, MD

The PROM King . . . 132
Mitchel A. Woltersdorf, PhD, PT

The Status of Occupational
Therapy in Canada . . . 133
Norman L. Burnette

Show Us Your Credentials . . . 134
Allen Mason

Fear of Flunking . . . 135
Charles DiMaggio, PA-C

Personal Reflections . . . 136
Tricia Hoare, RTNM

Why I Don't Teach
High School Chemistry . . . 137
Anonymous

"The Show Must Go On" . . . 138
Cecil Birtcher

Whose Balloon Is Expanding? . . . 139
Art Labelle, DDS

A History of Greece in One Page . . . 140
F. Clarke Fraser

A Look Back: History of Medicine . . . 140
Anonymous

WORD PLAY

Acronymitis, Anachroniphobia,
and Euphemismus . . . 143
David Wolman, PA-C

Soundings: Premedical Science . . . 144
George Dunea

The Doctor's Dictionary . . . 145
Howard J. Bennett, MD

The Venereal Game . . . 146
Francis V. Hanavan

Need a Chuckle?
Check Out These Codes . . . 147
Erno S. Daniel, MD

Fifty Ways to Love Your Liver
(With Apologies to Paul Simon) . . . 148
Jeffrey B. Moran

User-Friendly Microbiological
Nomenclature . . . 149
Edward M. Thompson, MD
Allen F. Shaughnessy, PharmD

Professionalism and Sono "Techs" . . . 150
Linda M. Chase, BA, BS, RDMS

Ridiculitis: More [sic] Humor . . . 151
John H. Dirckx, MD

Charting Chuckles . . . 152
Jan Black, RN, OCN

More Charting Chuckles . . . 153
Jan Black, RN, OCN

"RAAT": The Rehabilitation
Acronym and Abbreviation Test . . . 154
John Dolan, RhD
Ralph E. Matkin, RhD

An Educator Calls for a Standardization
of Terms: Taking the Fat Out of
Respiratory Care's Alphabet Soup . . . 155
Joseph G. Sorbello, MEd, RRT

WE'RE ALL IN THIS TOGETHER

New Yawk, New Yawk . . . 159
DEXTER HUNT, BA, EMT-P

Learning Experiences . . . 161
RENEA AKIN, MHS, PT

Ask Sirenhead . . . 162
SIRENHEAD

Prostates and Other Touchy Subjects . . . 163
THOMAS W. O'CONNOR, PHARMD, MBA

So Here's Another Valentine's Day . . . 164
KATHY NEPHEW
MARIBETH LEAHY

An EMS Christmas . . . 165
SHEILA DRAZIC

The Tech Who Mooed at a Surgeon . . . 166
MICHAEL RAMSEY, PHD, CLS(NCA), CLSPH(NCA)

The Perturbed Rattler . . . 167
GREG NELSON, EMT-P

So We Think We Are Unique . . . 169
MARY JENKINS

Absolutely Flabulous . . . 170
COLLEEN WEDDERBURN TATE

First Person . . . 171
BRENDAN SMITH, EMT-P

With Apologies to Andy Rooney . . . 173
DEXTER HUNT, BA, EMT-P

FAMILY FUNCTIONS

"So, Here It Is September Again . . . Let Me Tell You What I Did Last Summer." . . . 177
RUSSELL L. MALONE

Stardom's Lure . . . 178
BEN DICKINSON, PHARMD STUDENT

Put Down the Duckie . . . 179
ANN F. VANSANT, PHD, PT

The Male Midlife Crisis . . . 180
THEODORE E. KEATS, MD

The View Askew . . . 181
PAT VIETENTHAL, RN

Lessons in Dependency:
Advice from a Failure . . . 182
BOB DEMERS, BS, RRT

Of Cats, Dogs, and Drug Interactions . . . 183
PHILIP D. HANSTEN, PHARMD

Thanksgiving? . . . 184
MARY GRAYSON

The Folly of Family Vacations . . . 185
DAVE BARRY

The OT Spouse . . . 187
J. W. YEAGER

Book Bibliography . . . 189

Journal Bibliography . . . 191

Author Index . . . 197

ACKNOWLEDGMENTS

First and foremost, all the selected authors have benefited this volume by sharing their knowledge and creativity. Without exception, they were generous with reprint permissions and in some cases even suggested other material that they thought would be appropriate to include.

Phyllis Jayne Evans drew most of the drawings at the beginning of each chapter. She was a delight to work with and we were somehow able to share the same vision through using only e-mail and phone calls.

Ruth Marcolina, Spencer Marsh, Miriam Swank and other colleagues at the SUNY Stony Brook Health Sciences Center Library were lavish in their support. It's very unusual to work in such an encouraging environment with co-workers who were always on the lookout for potential sources of material.

My husband, Erwin London, and stepson Steven deserve thanks for tolerating very relaxed housekeeping standards along with healthy appetites for take-out dinners.

Anne Kirsch graciously allowed me to rummage throughout her hospital library collection.

Thanks are due to Dr. Hector Sepulveda for his encouragement and for never once asking if the book was done.

National Library of Medicine Collection Access Section staff were extremely helpful by providing unusual access to the collection.

The Professional Development and Quality of Working Life Committee of New York State/ United University Professions granted a research study leave that allowed time to freely pursue this project.

INTRODUCTION

This book is intended for all health professionals who are interested in enjoying a humorous moment, but especially for those in the allied health fields. More than a collection of articles, this book highlights common themes across all disciplines, expressing a collective understanding regardless of authors' occupational choices, and demonstrating that humor is a necessary part of their working lives.

The original intention was to seek out material only from the allied health fields as defined in the *AMA Health Professions Career and Education Directory*. Some of these fields include clinical laboratory technology, dental assistant, dietitian, emergency medical technician, occupational therapist, physical therapist, physician assistant, respiratory therapist, and surgical technologist. It was a difficult search for material in the health-related professional literature for a variety of reasons. These fields are relatively new compared to medicine and nursing, the published body of literature is small in many occupations, and perhaps they tend to take themselves too seriously in the process of establishing their reputation and gaining respect. The more traditional ways of locating material such as by using bibliographies, indexes, and database searches are of limited value since, from past experience, I learned that most humor is not effectively indexed. It was only by compiling lists of likely allied health journals and then scanning them page by page for the most recent ten years that most of the material was uncovered. As the search for materials continued and the months dragged on, some wonderful material in the medical and nursing literature was located and included if it had general appeal.

Not being a health care provider was an advantage as well as a disadvantage for deciding which material to include. Sources were viewed from an outsider's viewpoint, or one might say from a naïve perspective. Thus, it was difficult to always tell if the jargon was appropriate or if the humor would be understood by those in other fields. It occurred to me that since this was a collection from many different occupations, the reader would most likely be familiar with only one area of expertise. So if I understood a piece, it should be easy for others to appreciate. Another advantage in searching out material was that all disciplines and fields were of equal interest.

It must be readily admitted that the selection of articles was absolutely and totally subjective. Occasionally, I gave others material to evaluate if there was any question about inclusion. Sometimes my test subjects thought the material was very funny and I just didn't get it at all. A decision eventually had to be made, so in the final analysis, it was quality of the writing and interest of the subject matter that demonstrated the special nature of that occupation, while still not being so provincial that it would appeal only to members of that specialty, that were the deciding factors.

Items from 77 different journal titles have been selected, with only about one out of four articles that were originally thought to have potential being included. Of course, copyright permissions had to be obtained and some material was lost during this process. Every attempt was made to include only the best material according to my rather subjective criteria. In addition to being humorous, if a piece represented a profession that doesn't have much published humor and also addressed a recurrent motif, then it had a good chance of being chosen. It is true that after the fourth reading it is an extraordinary piece that can still make you laugh. The oldest article is from 1923 and it is truly amazing that some of the same issues of respect from colleagues and patients are being discussed today.

The eleven chapters are arranged according to common themes that all health care providers will likely experience. Media images of health care providers in movies, newspapers, radio, and television are first because this permeates our collective consciousness. "Today Might be Different" tells the straight story of what life is actually like on the inside. Describing daily events while taking care of patients is the subject of the next chapter. Of course, even health care providers occasionally get sick and need to trade places and become the patient. It's almost too easy to make fun of managed care, because along with vast changes have come plenty of absurdities. "What it Really Means" is about the various ways that the same incident may be seen by those who have learned to view life from more than one perspective. Management and supervision within the health care arena are next with proof that the best managers know their chains of command well, provide necessary resources, and then just get out of the way. That old saying about the more things change the more they remain the same is just as true for allied health fields. With so many abbreviations, acronyms, and jargon, we share a common language in "Word Play." This is followed by "We're All in This Together," which chronicles how prevalent and all-inclusive work experiences are for all allied health professionals. Finally, at the end of a long day, we go home and see how well our family functions with the demands of work.

Two bibliographies are included, one for recent book titles on benefiting from humor and the other for journal articles. The vast majority of books and articles have been published within the last ten years, with a tremendous amount of writing done in the last five years alone. Most of the material deals with learning how to effectively utilize humor with colleagues, patients, and students. One especially interesting section contains ways to improve your sense of humor, which it seems can be a learned skill just like any other.

In George Vaillant's *Adaptation to Life* he wrote, "Humor is one of the truly elegant defenses in the human repertoire. Few would deny that the capacity for humor, like hope, is one of mankind's most potent antidotes for the woes of Pandora's box." Perhaps by opening this book and releasing the gift of laughter, you will be empowered to let humor become your partner in practice.

Colleen Kenefick

IT'S NEWS TO ME

It seems like you can't watch TV, go to a movie, or read the newspaper anymore without encountering a health care professional. While not exactly staples on the evening news, they are invariably present at the latest natural or man-made disaster scene or shown in a lab participating in yet another medical breakthrough. It's no wonder that health care professionals are always fantasizing about being famous and having their moment in the spotlight. So, get in touch with your inner actor and see if being "discovered" could be in your future.

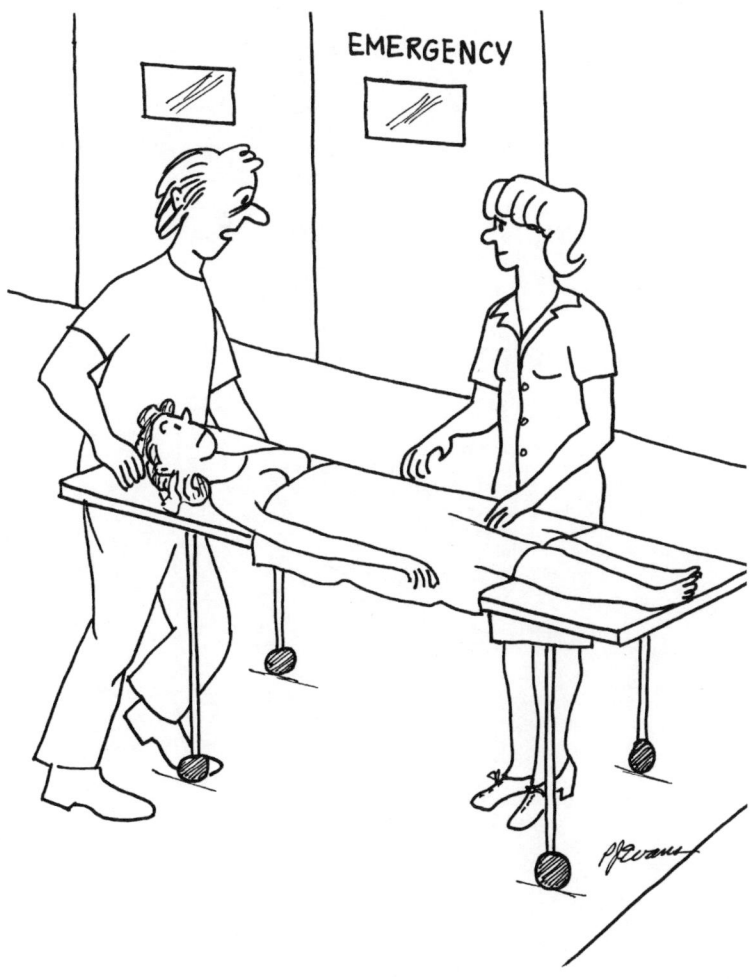

"If one more patient tells me how George Clooney would do it, I'll scream."

THE NEWS FROM LAKE MINDBEGONE

J. Russell Teagarden, MA

(Sponsored by Sam's Pretty Good Drug Store, where if you can't find it at Sam's, you'll probably find it at the Walgreen's down the street.)

Lake Mindbegone, God's little insane asylum, is a town on the eastern shore of Lake Mindbegone, in the farther reaches of civilization. No one knows whether the town took its name from the lake or whether the lake was named for the town. The entire populace of 633 is psychotic to various degrees, and all require treatment. In fact, when Lake Mindbegoners are referred to as tardy, it's not because they are late. No one is quite sure how it came to be that the entire town suffers from psychosis. The most recent theory has something to do with overexposure to video games.

Despite treatment with an assortment of drugs, electroconvulsive therapy, and frontal lobotomies, only a few Lake Mindbegoners can scratch out a living; the others must subsist on the benevolence of the state. Except on Sundays, when they are listening to Father Sane at Our Lady of Perpetual Donations, and except for frequent trips to the shore, many of the townspeople spend their time at the Psychobabble Cafe. It is usually rather quiet at the Psychobabble Cafe; not much to talk about. The nearby Spinal Tap Bar is also popular, but it is at the Psychobabble that most information, such as it is, gets exchanged. The information is generally provided by those few folks who have a semblance of a grip on things.

It was a typical Friday night at the Psychobabble Cafe recently when Daphne ("Daffy") Desyrel told about the release of a new drug that could revive the inhabitants of Lake Mindbegone. "The drug is called clozapine, and it's made by Sandoz," said Daffy excitedly.

This confused many at first, because "sand doze" is a local expression that refers to taking a nap at the beach, which most Lake Mindbegoners do at least twice a day. Quite a celebration ensued the next day, however. There was a big parade and a barbecue at the beach, and as darkness descended the Extrapyramidal Players began a concert. The celebration was dampened somewhat when Paula Parnate forgot about the dietary restrictions associated with her medication and died of a hypertensive crisis. An all too common occurrence at these town parties.

The following Monday, the townspeople rushed to the office of the visiting psychiatrist Naomi ("Dr. Normal") Navane (who would never live in Lake Mindbegone—too many crazy people) and asked her just to write the town a prescription and be done with it.

"No can do," said Dr. Normal to the crowd assembled before the little professional building.

"Why not?" exclaimed the Lake Mindbegoners.

"Because Sam's Pretty Good Drug Store isn't allowed to stock or dispense clozapine," replied Dr. Normal.

"Well, how about the Walgreen's down the street?"

"No, they can't either."

"Hmm . . . so much for Sam's motto," observed someone.

"You see," explained Dr. Normal, "no pharmacy can dispense or control this drug, not even hospital pharmacies."

"Jeez, what gives?" asked the townspeople.

"Well, there is an infrequent but dangerous adverse effect of clozapine that can result in death if not caught early. Therefore, blood samples must be drawn and reviewed weekly. Sandoz was able to talk the FDA into restricting access to this drug such that they see to the monitoring and distribute

Reprinted with permission from *American Journal of Hospital Pharmacy*, © 1990; 47(11):2536–2537.

it directly to patients through a home health-care company. They call this the Clozaril Patient Management System."

Ella Ville, who was benefiting from a recent dosage adjustment, said, "It sounds fishy to me, but what the hell, sign us up!"

"There's a hitch," said Dr. Normal, "about $9000 worth of hitch per person per year."

"Yikes," responded Ella, "Glad we're all on public aid."

"Oh yeah?" chuckled Normal. "The state says it's too expensive and won't pay for it. Plus, despite the whining of pharmacists around the country and letters from the FDA, Sandoz will not alter its stance. So all of you, like thousands of others in similar predicaments, are out of luck."

Pete O. Frane, who had not been heard to speak a word in over 35 years, piped up and captured the sentiments of the town: "That stinks!"

"You're so right, Pete," said Normal, "especially when you realize that people in other countries who need clozapine do not have to go through this system and spend this amount of money."

"Like Germany, maybe?" asked Daffy.

"For one," replied Normal. "Why do you mention Germany?"

Daffy squared her shoulders and addressed everyone: "Well, my brother Mel is visiting there right now. Perhaps he could bring a load of clozapine home!"

Dr. Normal put on a long face, but finally she smiled. "OK, sounds good. Get the boy on the blower."

Daffy negotiated the international telephone system, and Mel generously consented to make the haul, although he could not say when.

Mel had become involved with a Bavarian named Gertrude. The relationship persisted for several months after Daffy's call. Gertrude eventually dumped Mel when he started spending more time talking to himself than to her. Mel went into a tailspin but eventually got hold of himself. He also got hold of an airplane ticket and a sackful of the clozapine that would save Lake Mindbegone.

All went well until Mel reached customs at Kennedy International Airport. He felt more disturbed than usual when he approached the customs officer with the pressed uniform and shiny name tag ("Jack Range" was engraved on it). And as it turned out, Mel had good reason to feel uneasy. Officer Jack Range was all over him like white on rice and quickly discovered the contraband.

"This stuff looks like clozapine," accused Jack.

"It is," confessed Mel. "How did you know?"

"I happen to be an undercover agent for Sandoz," said Jack. "We expected that people would be trying to smuggle this stuff in."

"Oops," muttered Mel.

"What are you, crazy?" asked Jack.

"Why, yes."

"Don't you know about the Clozaril Patient Management System?" asked an indignant Jack.

"Maybe a little," replied Mel, "but only from reading banal messages posted on electronic bulletin boards by some jerk in Chicago."

"You've got enough clozapine in here to treat a small town," said Jack.

"That's the idea, I'm told."

"You're in big trouble, pal," snarled Jack. "Obtaining and using clozapine in any fashion not specified by the package labeling can be interpreted as a violation of the Food, Drug and Cosmetic Act. I'm taking you downtown. First we'll check your white blood cell count. If it's low, we'll send you back to Germany. If it's normal, we prosecute—immediately!"

Mel was yearning for Gertrude and maybe a Wiener schnitzel.

The townspeople of Lake Mindbegone never found out what became of Mel (in fact, he wound up in San Quentin). They could only hope that one day clozapine would be freely available to them and others in need of it. They haunted the Psychobabble Cafe and held out their hope in disjointed sentences.

That's all the news from Lake Mindbegone, where all the women are clinically depressed, all the men are crazy, and all the children are learning disabled.

TABLOID MEDICINE AND THE MEDICAL OPTIONS MARKET

David Wolman, PA-C

There is much confusion among the public about medicine these days, not only about health care reform—which, by virtue of Newt, now resembles a chunk of ice onto which the sick and weak will be kindly floated out to sea—but also about disease itself.

What I mean is that many major issues in health maintenance have become like the options market. One day something is good for you, the next day it isn't; if you don't unload that freight car of treadmills and HDLs quickly, you'll be stuck with a bad deal because you missed the next wave of medical advances, corrections, and contradictory findings. No wonder Captain Kirk went from selling Promise Margarine to "Rescue 911."

My medical education needs are now in part met by reading a mix of the lay press, supermarket tabloids, women's magazines, and health magazines, and by viewing such edifying shows as "20/20" and "Primetime Live"—not to mention "ER" and "Chicago Hope." How else would I know that pediatric care in emergency departments is inferior? That Ebola virus is among us? That doctors overprescribe antibiotics? That necrotizing fasciitis chews off your arm so fast you don't realize it until you go to brush your teeth....

Physicians don't, unfortunately, watch this stuff. In fact, many medical breakthroughs I read about are unknown to doctors. An article in the *New York Times* recently, for example, reported that researchers had isolated the substance that large tumors exude to inhibit vascularization in metastatic lesions. If this substance can be manufactured, the article said, trials may begin with a potent weapon against cancer.

Well, I spoke to two oncologists, both respected in their fields, and neither of them had heard about this finding. And they both assured me that this was not unusual, because very often the first news they hear about a medical advance comes from a patient.

Medical journals don't, as a group, always seem very coherent, either. I perused several recently; as an example of my point, here are risk factors for breast cancer based on findings in three recent articles in three publications:

- Increasing age (by 50 years, chances are 1 in 50)
- High-fat diet
- Staying *out* of the sun
- High caloric intake
- Low intake of β-carotene
- Alcohol (but alcohol may lower your risk of heart disease)
- The pesticide DDT
- Family history
- Benign breast disease (it makes exams and mammograms less effective)
- Late age at first childbirth
- Early menarche
- Higher education and socioeconomic status (but this helps you afford all that β-carotene and vacations in the sun)
- Decreased exercise
- Western culture
- Exogenous estrogen
- Interrupted first pregnancy
- Psychosomatic factors.

What's a woman to do? Become a poor, young, vegetarian, sun-worshiping, teetotaling, uneducated mother having a slew of babies at 17? Is the sum of information produced by medical journals, the press, and television in proportion to society's confusion, mistrust, and noncompliance? Maybe.

This gave me an idea. As physician assistants, we obviously have more time to keep up with advances in medicine through the medium of popular culture. I say we have more time because, unlike physicians, we don't spend most of our waking

Reprinted with permission from Journal of the American Academy of Physician Assistants, © 1995; 8(4):21–22.

hours figuring out how to play the managed care game. We practice medicine and go home. Plenty of time to read *People* and watch Barbara Walters. So perhaps a new role for us is to take the initiative as popularizers of medicine.

It isn't, after all, reassuring when your doctor doesn't know what you are talking about when you mention the epidemic of "walking pneumonia" reported recently in your local gazette. But if we PAs peruse the popular media, we can step in and say: "Yeah, I read about that—right next to the article on the Elvis sighting. Walking pneumonia is something we are vigilant against. We hate to see anybody walk around with anything. *Especially* pneumonia. On the other hand, we don't want to create one of those multiply drug-resistant bacteria that just destroyed Cleveland. As reported in *Power Rangers Weekly*."

We live in a world where medical news is big business. Every television news program now has a medical segment. Alternative medicine is a $3-billion-a-year business. Information has become so voluminous, so available, and so contradictory that we may have become the smartest ignoramuses in history. Every time I suggest pursuing a treatment or prescribing a drug, someone chimes in with a recent finding from some questionable source that challenges the wisdom of my cure. There is so much clatter of medical talk out there that we are paralyzed with an abundance of nonsense.

Getting back to my main point: Because we are not doctors, we can create a sense of camaraderie with our patients. We can help them to sort through the trees to get to the forest. And, in doing so, we need not scoff at them. We can be open to folk remedies, rumors, and fears, and can try to guide our patients into a better understanding of how *relative* everything is. In 99% of cases, less is more; we can make our patients happy and tell them not to let Geraldo spoil their sense of wellness. On the other hand, we should tell them that if they are truly sick, they can trust tried-and-true cures. They do not need a laparoscopic wart removal; liquid nitrogen may do the trick. And stay away from toads.

I think PAs should be reading more *Elle* and less *JAMA*, more *Prevention* and less *New England Journal of Medicine*, to bridge the gap between the so-called scientific journals and the so-called lay media. We are in the perfect position to be communicators, interpreters of the debris-littered information highway.

Let's be responsible for our patients' health, to the best of our knowledge and ability. But let's not ignore medical UFOs; we should reassure patients that, wherever these aliens are from, it can't be as confusing a place as earth, and that as soon as the creatures watch one episode of "Sixty Minutes," they'll be outta here. At warp speed.

INSTRUCTIONS FOR EDITORS:

A "Revenge Fantasy"
Joseph Herman

In his "Psychopathology of Everyday Life," Freud speaks of experiencing a "revenge phantasy."

I, too, have a revenge fantasy. It concerns the editors and reviewers who have cracked the whip of rejection and revision over me for 30 years. The balance of power between them, who could not exist without authors, and authors who would not have to exist were there no journals, urgently needs redressing and my fantasy runs like this: An Authors' Collaboration is being formed to deal with editors on an equal footing and there is even talk of a boycott. Each member has been asked what he or she finds most irksome in the author/editor relationship. Because I wrote down "Instructions for Authors," I have been asked to look into the possibility of compiling a set of "Instructions for Editors" with which any journal wishing to receive submissions from the Collaboration will have to comply. Knowing how to reference the Book of Job or "Hamlet" correctly does wonders for the ego and will, no doubt, be of much use in my future writing.

I have been at work on Instructions for Editors for some time and what ensues consists of only a few salient examples; the finished document will have a reading time of 40 minutes. My own comments are in parentheses after the rulings.

Review Process

1B: An editorial decision must be handed down within 48 hours of the arrival of a submission. If this requirement is not met, the Collaboration or any of its members may refer the manuscript to another journal. (This rule saves considerable effort and expense by dispensing with the need for a letter of acknowledgment.)

1C: The outside of the envelope containing the editor's decision must be stamped either A for acceptance or R for rejection. (This precaution is intended to prevent undue prolongation of the Q-T (query/tear) interval with possible serious consequences for an aspiring author.)

1F: Letters of rejection must be typed, double-spaced with four-inch margins all around, even in countries where the metric system obtains. They must not contain any statistics on acceptance rates or statements to the effect that rejection does not necessarily reflect on the submission's quality. If the editor feels constrained to transmit a reviewer's comments—"You may find them useful in seeking publication elsewhere"—he or she must make sure they contain no more than one ad hominem remark. (Such venting of spleen allows the remainder to come to the point.) The recommended wording for a letter of rejection is as follows:

> Dear Dr...
>
> Thank you for your submission to our journal. It is by far the best piece of research we have ever received. Unfortunately, the editorial board has just committed itself to publishing a study on the same subject of vastly inferior design but with similar outcome. We have no doubt that your paper will soon elicit a favorable response from another journal, hopefully with an impact factor as high as ours.
>
> Sincerely (but not yours)

Submission of Letters

2A: Send an original and four high quality copies to the corresponding author at the following addresses which he or she will provide: home, place of work, accountant, golf or tennis club, eldest daughter's piano teacher. The envelope may not be franked but must bear postage stamps from among those most recently issued in the country of origin, at least one for every author. Picturesque stamps will be given

---

Reprinted from Journal of Clinical Epidemiology, © 1998; 51(6): 525–526, with permission from Elsevier Science. Edited from the original.

preference and will bring about a more rapid handling of editorial correspondence.

References

3B: No journal continuing to subscribe to the "et al." rule—six authors or editors referenced, the rest subsumed under "et al."—will receive submissions from the Collaboration. All authors or editors must be named in every reference. ("Et al.," according to the dictionary, means "and others." This becomes an absurdity if there are precisely seven persons who should be named since the single one omitted cannot be referred to in the plural. For example, Dr. Richard K. Root is the seventh editor of the 12th edition of "Harrison's Principles of Internal Medicine" and so is the only one to be left out when the book is quoted. I have tried to slip him past the regulation, but either the paper in question was rejected or I was caught out. Whatever the case, he owes me a word of gratitude and I expect to hear from him shortly.)

Denouement

Freud "awoke" from his daydream of revenge in the following manner: "At this point my phantasy was interrupted by a loud 'Good evening, Professor!' and as I looked up, there was the same couple on whom I had just taken this imaginary vengeance." My awakening consists of stepping down into the street for a breath of fresh air and noticing an official-looking envelope in my mailbox. It contains a letter from the editor of a journal whose pages I have been trying to crash for years. The first line reads: "We are pleased to inform you. . . ." I have tendered my resignation to the Collaboration!

HOW TO KILL AN ASSOCIATION

Don't participate beyond paying your dues—let "them" handle things.
Then complain that members have no voice in management.
Decline all offices and committee appointments—you're too busy.
Then offer vociferous advice on how they should do things.
If appointed to a committee, don't work—it's a courtesy appointment.
Then complain because the organization has stagnated.
If you do attend management meetings, don't initiate new ideas.
Then you can play "Devil's Advocate" to those submitted by others.

Don't rush to pay your dues—they're too high anyway.
Then complain about poor financial management.
Don't encourage others to become members—that's selling.
Then complain that membership is not growing.
Don't read the mail from headquarters—it's not important.
Then complain that you're not kept informed.
Don't volunteer your talents—that's ego fulfillment.
Then complain that you're never asked; never appreciated.
And, if by chance, the organization grows in spite of your contributions. . .
Grasp every opportunity to tell the youngsters how tough it was; how hard you worked in the old days to bring the organization to its present level of success.

Reprinted from Dental Assistant, © 1980; 49(4):5, with permission from the Virginia Academy of Family Physicians.

A DIFFERENT KIND OF TURF BATTLE

Jules M. Rothstein, PhD, PT

Disconcerting news of a bizarre new turf battle has come in from the United Kingdom. American physical therapists are no strangers to turf battles over professional prerogatives, but I have never heard of a case like this one. At the University of East Anglia, plans for new facilities for physiotherapy and occupational therapy are being jeopardized by previous claims to the building site, an abandoned golf course. Apparently, a group of squatters have had long-term residency on the site. To make matters worse, there is documented evidence that the squatters are capable of fierce and savage behavior; in fact, they spend most of their time fighting and killing each other. Although it may be hard to believe, it appears that in the land of Beatrix Potter and Peter Rabbit, there is a bunny equivalent to the Manson family.

Ensconced on the old golf course is a vast rabbit warren. For seven years, two East Anglian animal behaviorists have made careers out of documenting the dark side of the rabbit world. These biologists now fear that their living laboratory will be plowed under. But university officials, who claim the biologists were given due notice, have decreed that, in 1991, when the biologists' grants end, the golf course and the rabbits must give way to new buildings. Any researcher would feel sympathetic to these well-respected biologists, but, then again, perhaps the biologists should look on the bright side of things. These particular biologists have been documenting the truly horrendous behavior of killer rabbits. As one of the biologists has noted, even the babies lack civility: You can see "balls of fluff at six weeks beating the hell out of one another" (Science 246:1384, 1989). The future seems even more dismal; the biologists report that the proportion of the most dominant and vicious rabbits is increasing.

If the rabbits must go, and it appears that they must, the biologists should consider the possibilities. The university wants to build student dormitories and physiotherapy and occupational therapy facilities on the site. Now, that is grist for animal behaviorists. Consider the observations that could be made in that environment.

I hope our colleagues in East Anglia get their new building. I wish the biologists well in their new endeavors. But as for the rabbits? As one of the biologists has said, "They're not . . . *Watership Down* characters who simply pack their bags and move to pastures new." Amen! The thought of killer rabbits spreading throughout the English countryside evokes frightening images of bloody turf battles. As we approach the season of the Easter Bunny, let's hope that more peaceable rabbits prevail, and that we can all put turf battles behind us.

Reprinted from Physical Therapy, © 1990; 70(3):149, with the permission of the APTA.

TRY IGNORANCE

Gabor B. Levy

The report that "America is Becoming a Nation of Culture" (*Wall Street Journal*, Sept. 17, 1998) was encouraging. The article proved the claim by statistics showing that, e.g., in 1997 fully 35% of the people visited museums at least once, versus 22% in 1982, that in the same time span twice the number of students got credit for studies abroad, and that 41% of people listened to "classical" music compared to 19% earlier. It also cited the doubling of wine consumption and a large increase in fine-dining establishments, but this seems to indicate affluence rather than culture. I took a stab at it myself, and found that about 2½ times as many nonfiction books are borrowed from the Westport, Connecticut, Public Library than mysteries and other books of fiction. This is in sharp contrast to the horrific figures reported by the International Center of Scientific Literacy. It found that only 11% of those queried could define "molecule," half believed that dinosaurs and humans coexisted at one time, and only 48% knew that the earth orbits the sun once a year. Galileo died over 350 years ago, and he must be turning in his grave.

Trying to reconcile such opposing data leads to the realization that although there may indeed be more wine-sipping museum-goers, the bulk of the population is ill-informed. Although America has probably the most erudite scholars in many fields, we may be facing a parallel situation as in incomes, where the rich get richer and the poor get poorer. An inescapable conclusion must be that the educational establishment is at fault. There have been many complaints about the defects in education, and many suggestions on how to remedy them. But few if any point to the root of the problem, which is the basic principle on which it currently rests. It is that everybody is equally educatable. It is this false and entirely novel doctrine that colors everything. It is rigidly held, despite thousands of years of experience, that people are not equally able to absorb knowledge. An illustrative anecdote from 15th-century Italy refers to the great clock, whose ringing and single hand showed the hours to all people while the phases of the moon and other astronomical subtleties were displayed *"agli intelligenti,"* for the educated.

Ancillary to the fallacy that everybody must be equally educatable is that you can *teach* any subject. Actually, beyond simple drills like the multiplication tables and quasifunctional literacy, most subjects cannot be taught. The teacher's job in these instances is, substantially, to guide and help students to learn. There is a huge difference in these concepts, because you can help only those who are receptive. Motivation is everything.

In the face of this reality, our current educational establishment persists in maintaining the fiction of universal educability. In order to be able to boast an 82% graduation rate from high school, as compared to about only one-third of the population in 1950, and to have 23.6% obtain college degrees, as compared to 6.2% at the earlier date, the curricula have simply been diluted and made more superficial. I was astonished when my granddaughter, a student at a first-class eastern university, took such filler courses to complete the necessary credits for graduation. One was "Wine Appreciation" and another "Science Fiction and Physical Phenomena." This does not seem to be exceptional. I scanned the program of a community college and found such courses as #255: "The Language of Seduction," #325: "Gender in Architecture," #593b: "Intimate Relations," and #594a: "Psychology of Eating and Drinking," while a New York high school offered a credit course in making graffiti. Such intellectual dilution reaches far and wide. There is a new Girl Scout badge on shopping called "Fashion Adventure." Even physical education is not immune, and has become "Physical Focus." Calisthenics is abandoned in favor of games like playing tag with rubber chickens.

These observations relate to the United States, but they may be applicable globally, perhaps spreading

---

Reprinted with permission from American Laboratory, © 1999; 31(6):6,8. Edited from the original.

in the shadow of democracy. Theodore Darymple, in an editorial in the *Wall Street Journal* (December 9, 1998), said that in his area of an English industrial city he called a slum, he found that "Only one of the hundreds of teenagers knew when World War II was fought." "The name of Shakespeare sometimes rings faint bells, sometimes not." ". . . even the answer to such sums as 9 plus 12 often eludes them. Two have given me the answer 20, and when I told them that it was nearly right, but not quite . . . they smiled happily at their unexpected success." Darymple, who is a physician rather than an educator, concluded his essay with this provocative observation: "When young people between 16 and 20 are given cognitive tests administered to old people to discover whether they are suffering from dementia, a high proportion of the youngsters are found already suffering from mental deficiency. English schools give you Alzheimer's."

The abandonment of basic courses that seem tedious at times has consequences transcending the lack of knowledge. In my school days we had virtually no choices, and in engineering school, where some elective cultural courses were offered, they did not count toward a degree. We had to study a lot of things of only marginal use in our careers. But they served to teach us discipline and the techniques of finding and organizing knowledge. It also prepared us for the fact that in adult life you must put up with some tedium in order to reach your goals. In the current trends to make studies "fun" and easy, students get a distorted picture of adult existence. There can be lots of pleasure in work, but it comes at a price. Every discovery has to be validated by boring repetition, and challenged even at the danger of disappointment. These vital lessons are lost today.

We cannot blame our educational system for all social ills. Still, much blame must rest on the educational establishment that produces so many half-educated, gullible, self-indulgent, and socially dysfunctional young adults. The guiding principle in education seems to have become—to paraphrase a statement of the former president of Harvard University. If learning is too onerous, try ignorance!

THAT'S ENTERTAINMENT

Neal A. Whitman, EdD

After having himself committed for suicidal urges to a mental institution, Hunter "Patch" Adams discovers that his clowning around has a good effect on himself and other patients and decides to go to medical school, where he defies the dean and proves that laughter is the best medicine. The closing credits tell us that the Gesundheit Institute, a free clinic started by Patch and fellow students, treated 15,000 patients and had a waiting list of 1,000 physicians offering their services. Apparently, in real life, the clinic fell on hard times, so Patch wrote a book about his story, got movie offers, and ta-da! Robin Williams has taken on the screen role.

The movie drives home a point well-known to medical educators: yes, it is hard for medical students to keep their humanity. One dean put it this way at freshman orientation: "You arrive wanting to do good and leave wanting to do well." While there probably are medical schools now eager to have Dr. Adams visit and tell his story in person, his portrayal in the movie bugged me. Here are the 10 reasons why:

#10. Patch enters medical school and graduates in 1971, the same year I began my career in academic medicine. In my experience, medical schools were not immune from the social revolution of the

Reprinted with permission of the author and Perspective on Physician Assistant Education, © 1999; 10(1):44–45. Edited from the original.

1960s and the curriculum by then already had made room for the doctor-patient relationship. You would never know that from the movie, which portrays the entire faculty as "aloof, arrogant, and devoid of any vision of humane health care."

#9. If Patch is such a great humanitarian, why is he shown falling in love with the best-looking woman in his class, rather than the warmest, most caring? The actress Monica Potter is cute as a button and Patch is smitten before she says a word.

#8. Patch is shocked, shocked, shocked to find out that 2 years of basic science instruction precede clinical clerkships. Of course, this is the same college freshman who admitted himself to a mental institution where he was shocked, shocked, shocked to discover that he would not be housed in a private room. Doesn't Patch look before he leaps? In his book, he admits that when he entered the Medical College of Virginia in 1967, "I didn't know much about medicine; I just expected to become a doctor without realizing what that meant."

#7. In his first year, Patch decides to make his own hospital rounds, cruising in and out of patients' rooms, telling jokes, and pulling stunts. He knows nothing about the patients and their families, never mind their medical conditions. We see little listening, but much performing. So much for two-way communication.

#6. Patch's repeated defiance of rules leads to visits to both the academic dean's and the executive dean's offices—all mahogany, dimly lit—too dark to read a budget report. I've met some pretty starched medical school administrators in my time, but the executive dean is beyond belief ... and why can't Patch keep a promise?

#5. Patch and fellow students start a free clinic somewhere overlooking the Blue Ridge Mountains, stocked with stolen hospital supplies. They treat patients with no medical supervision, which, if true, sounds pretty dangerous to me. I tip my hat to Utah medical students who staff a homeless clinic in Salt Lake City where supervisory faculty also volunteer—in fact, students and faculty across the U.S. collaborate all the time in charitable efforts.

#4. Patch's medical school roommate-grind, the stereotyped "son of a son of a son of a doctor," converts to Patch's humanitarian approach to medicine after Patch's love interest (see #9) is murdered by a psychotic free-clinic patient. The shotgun murder-suicide only proves that Patch and his fellow unsupervised students were out of their league.

#3. When Patch is finally kicked out of medical school for practicing medicine without a license (duhh), his appeal to the state board of medical examiners is held in a medical school lecture hall filled to the rafters with students ... but not an attorney in sight. And, bringing in the cancer kids to show their support was pretty pathetic.

#2. Patch insults the appeals board and they reward him by deciding that Medicine needs fresh air. Speaking of fresh air, Patch rewards the same board that reinstated him by mooning them at his medical school graduation. Pulease.

#1. This movie fit into the *One Flew Over the Cuckoo's Nest* genre of movies pioneered by Miles Forman and Jack Nicholson and now championed by Robin Williams: Just let crazy people run the world and we'll be better off.

To be fair, Patch's personal history, told in the introduction to his book, *Gesundheit*, is a little different from the one told in the movie. In real life, he met his wife in the last weeks of medical school, not on the first day. And, although he did work in a free clinic during his senior year, he did not start his own clinic until he quit Georgetown's pediatric residency ... the murder of his true love by a deranged patient apparently was just a ploy to sensationalize the movie.

DANGER IN THE NEWSROOM

Kevin Shea O'Malley, RPh

Some pharmacists are high-strung, but 30 years of running Doug's Drugs had left Douglas Codger wound tighter than an eight-day clock. The poor sap trembled like a Chihuahua on Dexedrine from the moment he entered my office.

"Lex Icon, special investigator?" He managed to get the words out between paroxysms.

"Just like it says on the door," I allowed, motioning him to a chair while I rummaged around my desk for an alprazolam to give him for his nerves. I struck a match, then, after a moment's hesitation, opted for a Nicorette instead. "What can I do for you?" I asked as he took a seat.

Codger babbled on for some time about "that cheap rag" and "those sleazeball reporters" who he said were ruining his business, before I realized he was talking about *The Daily Prattler*.

The Prattler was one of those two-bit scandal sheets everyone reads while standing in the Food World checkout line, but no one buys unless they're pretty sure no one is looking. Anyway, last I had heard, *The Prattler*'s "Public Defenders" team was dashing around motel rooms with white gloves and black lights trying to uncover the latent dangers of motel-room mildew. It seemed pretty lame to me, but I figured that's what they had to do to sell papers.

Lucky for me, the benzodiazepine reached steady-state levels in about 20 minutes, and Codger started making a little sense. *The Prattler* apparently figured mildew wasn't dramatic enough and decided to make the small evolutionary leap up from fungi to pharmacists. According to Codger, their m.o. consisted of sending reporters with hidden cameras into local pharmacies. There, they presented fake prescriptions for a pair of drugs with a small likelihood of interacting—say, Vasotec and Dyazide—in hopes of catching pharmacists in flagrante delicto.

Most pharmacists, of course, realized the significance of such an interaction was just about nil, and that the physicians would be monitoring the patient's potassium levels. They decided to forgo discussion of the matter so they could give their attention to more urgent problems, such as controlling crowds, not collapsing, and using a microscope to read NDC numbers. Nevertheless, *The Prattler* ran a cover story accusing pharmacists of "blowing it" by overlooking "risky and even deadly drug interactions." What struck me as ironic was that, considering all the other problems plaguing this high-stress, low-profit, rapid-burnout profession (pharmacy, I mean, not journalism), *The Prattler* chose to concentrate on something of such minor importance. Sure, pharmacists occasionally make mistakes, but they rarely have anything to do with interactions, I thought.

Codger begged me to take the case. It seemed his nasty habit of signing cost-minus third-party contracts had already gotten him in Dutch, and all the bad press was putting the kibosh on his bottom line. He wanted me to dig up some dirt on the paper to discredit it, and thereby take people's mind off the pharmacy exposé. I thought it was the most harebrained scheme I'd ever heard, and was about to give him the bum's rush, when he asked if I'd ever heard of the tabloid's publisher, (the man who Codger believed carried a personal vendetta against pharmacists), Rupert Tubman.

My blood turned to ice water. Rupert Tubman, a.k.a. The Fat Man. At a hundred-fifty kilos, Tubman looked more like a poster child for the phen-fen diet than king of the tabloids. Back when I was teaching English at City College, about 10 years ago, we'd had a disagreement over syntax at a symposium. Tubman had had a couple of his goons drag me out in the alley during the break to do the Macarena on my kneecaps. That's when I decided teaching was too dicey for my blood and opened this business. I've been working Language Enforcement ever since, investigating everything from small-time grammar violations to felony cases of word abuse. Not only had I heard of Tubman, I

Reprinted with permission of the author and American Druggist, © 1997; 214(6):50–51.

thought about that corpulent creep every time I had to pop a Lodine XL to climb a flight of stairs.

I flashed Douglas Codger my best two-hundred-dollars-a-day-plus-expenses smile: "Call me Lex."

I figured my best bet at *The Prattler* was to turn the tables on them and go undercover myself in an attempt to ferret out mistakes early in manuscript production, before Spell-Check, before editors had a chance to clean things up. I submitted a fake resume, called in a couple favors, and in no time had myself a job as a janitor, armed with a hidden camera concealed in a mop bucket. Violations were everywhere; here's a sample of what I found in the first rough draft I looked at:

Offense	Number of Occurrences
Dangling participles	9
Split infinitives	5
Mixed tenses/Misplaced modifiers	7
Lack of subject and verb agreement	6
Spelling and punctuation errors	TMTC (too many to count)

I could go on. Sentence fragments were strewn all over the place. Reporters used "like" when they meant "as," and vice-versa. They ended sentences with prepositions. (I'm not about to.) They used far too many cliches, when everybody knows they're old hat.

Even now, thinking about what I saw at *The Prattler* nearly works me into a hypertensive crisis. Not that I mind when journalists exaggerate, misquote, take things out of context, fail to double-check facts, sensationalize, commit libel and destroy the lives of good people for the sake of a headline. Heck, I figure they have to do that stuff to make their stories interesting. What gets me hot under the collar is seeing how these journalists mangle the mother tongue I love so much. You ask me, they understand grammatical nuances about like I understand the significance of drug interactions occurring between macrolide antibiotics and nonsedating antihistamines metabolized via the cytochrome P450 mono-oxygenase system.

When I went public with my findings, newspaper industry representatives initially denied any wrongdoing. Then, when they realized I had 'em dead to rights, journalists argued that intense competition in their "increasingly unprofitable industry" and "pressure to meet deadlines" had turned their offices into sweatshops. They became contrite, saying how my report would give reporters a badly needed "wake-up call" and help to promote "badly needed change" in the industry. What do I think? I'll believe it when I see it.

My investigation was the beginning of the end for *The Prattler:* last week they filed for Chapter 13 bankruptcy protection, and it looks like the only thing Tubman will be publishing for some time will be the prison newsletter at the state correctional facility. Douglas Codger was vindicated, and who knows, Doug's Drugs may even turn a profit one day. (Provided, of course, he can steer clear of those third-party suicide contracts.)

I know a lot of people will say Language Enforcement is overrated. They'll say I'm a purist, and words don't matter, because after all, they're only marks on paper. Not me. I know better. I'm Lex Icon—and words is my life.

NIETZSCHE AND THE EVENING NEWS

Steven Tiger, PA

The late Dr. Robert Mendelsohn, pediatrician-author of *Confessions of a Medical Heretic* and other anti-medical establishment polemics, complained loudly and frequently that medicine had become a religion in this nation. He and his followers (disciples?) likened physicians to priests, medical school to seminary, hospitals to temples, and Medicalese to liturgical Latin. Certainly, the religious parallel is strengthened when we read in the literature that animals used in some laboratory experiment were "sacrificed."

Is there substance in this concept or doth the doctor protest too much? Is medicine a religion? Does our society worship medicine, looking to physicians for miracles and salvation? Considering how often the media use the phrase "medical miracle," how many people, if asked to name a miracle, would cite something related to medicine? Indeed, the media play a large role in fostering these attitudes.

No News Is Good News

The media have a strange relationship with medicine. The same hard-nosed reporters and commentators who ask tough questions when dealing with politicians, industrialists, and military leaders become suddenly sweet and docile when interviewing anyone in the medical establishment. Haven't we all seen this kind of story on the evening news?

CLOSE-UP OF ANCHORMAN: "... And now, here's Barbie, with tonight's 'Moment in Medicine.' Barbie?"

CUT TO BARBIE: "Thanks, Ken. In an article appearing in this month's issue of the *Journal of the American Obfuscatory Society*, Doctor So-and-so, head of the Department of Esotericology from the University of Such-and-such, has announced that this-and-that phenomenon may possibly, in certain circumstances, be related to some other thing. I interviewed Doctor So-and-so this morning, and here's a portion of what he said."

CUT TO VIDEOTAPE OF DR SO-AND-SO IN A WHITE COAT, SITTING BEHIND A DESK: "... Of course, Miss Doll, we'll need several more years of research before we can say whether or not these findings may someday lead to a new understanding of this question. But we're excited by the preliminary data."

BACK TO THE STUDIO, CLOSE-UP OF BARBIE: "Well, there you have it. A vital discovery that affects all of us. This 'Moment in Medicine' has been brought to you by Petro-Chem Pharmaceuticals, makers of Kitchensink® Kold-Kaps. Now back to you, Ken...."

Lots of the medical news reported by the popular media are comparably meaningless. What was that story about? A possible correlation that may or may not be valid or significant, and definitely won't have any clinical applicability for a considerable time, blown up out of proportion to its real meaning. There was no news at all in that story, but it became good news. The world may be choking in filth, the economy may be a shambles, and society may be disintegrating—but medicine offers Hope. Otherwise, the reporter's approach would be different: "Doctor, I understand that this study cost the taxpayers over three million dollars over the past two years. In view of the inadequacy of health care services in many parts of the nation, how can you justify spending so much public money on a project that may interest you intellectually but affects only a tiny percentage of the population?" But no!

So is it the media's fault? In part, yes. And what about Dr So-and-so? Asked about the story on television, he says, "Oh, no, I can't control how the

Reprinted from Physician Assistant, © 1991; 15(4):8,13, with permission of the author.

media read and report on what appears in the medical literature." Sure you can, doctor. When Barbie arrived to interview you, you could have said, "Listen, you twit, my research has no significance to anyone but a scientist right now, and it may come to nothing. If your audience is interested in what I have to say about health and medicine, tell them I said there are no miracles, and if they want to feel better, they should stop smoking, stop drinking and taking drugs, stop stuffing themselves with fat, sugar and salt, turn off the television, and start exercising." You could have said those things, doctor, but you didn't.

Doctor Shows

The news media are only part of the problem. Even Dr. So-and-so wasn't as impressive as the characters on medical soap-operas. You know the kind—square-jawed Chief of Surgery, saves 10 people before lunch, solves a murder and does community social work in the afternoon, then romances the heroine in the evening. Eventually, the writers realized they had to make their characters seem more human, more believable—so they gave them some lovable eccentricities. It's still God, but now God wears a funny hat.

Take this actual scene from a short-lived series called "Rafferty," about an eccentric neurologist. Rafferty is attending a concert, watching as a famous virtuoso performs a violin concerto. The performance is dazzling, the audience erupts in applause—and Rafferty rushes backstage to ask if the musician has been dropping things recently. He had noticed that the virtuoso used some unorthodox fingering in a certain difficult passage in the concerto, and correctly suspected a neurologic disorder.

Where do writers get such ideas? More important, how do such ideas affect people's thinking? And before you say there is no effect, remember that many people confuse actors and actresses with the characters they play on television. How much easier it is to confuse the general nature of the character with reality!

A Protest

Small wonder that people think of medicine as a superior world inhabited by superior beings. Someone is saying, "Hogwash, my patients certainly don't worship me." The fact that individual patients don't worship an individual medical practitioner doesn't preclude widespread public worship of the field of medicine.

Several years ago, a minister from a sociopolitically liberal church commented on the question of abortion. He said he prayed for the day when doctors would be able to define when a fetus becomes a person. Whatever your views on abortion, think about what it means for a clergyman to pray that doctors will resolve the matter.

Nietzsche was wrong. God isn't dead—He just went to medical school.

LETTER FROM AMERICA:

Quis Custodiet Ipsos Custodes?
Stuart A. Bentley

We all look forward to our 15 minutes of fame. Mine came a few weeks ago, but was not a source of unbridled joy. I serve on an expert panel of the Food and Drug Administration which met last August to review two new automated instruments for cervical cytology. The activities of the FDA are considered important politically and, in the interests of open government, meetings of its various expert panels are open to the public, including the press. Certain comments I made during the August meeting were picked up by an Associated Press reporter and disseminated through the wire service. What I actually said was that the new technology would not revolutionize cancer detection, but was a significant evolutionary advance. I distinctly remember the words I used, as I chose them carefully and thought they sounded rather good. The story subsequently found its way into several newspapers, including such heavy hitters as the *Washington Post* and the *New York Times*, where —to my chagrin—I was quoted as saying that the new technology "will not revolutionize things, it will evolutionize them."

Now, to the best of my knowledge, there is no such word as "evolutionize." If such a word were to exist, I would have no idea what it meant and whatever the case, it is far too ugly and cumbersome a word to find a place in my vocabulary. But the damage was already done. For several weeks, I had to endure the taunts of colleagues, who would point fingers at me, attach the "ize" suffix to an appropriate noun and then roll about in fits of uncontrollable laughter. "Could I come over to the laboratory and examinationize a bone marrow?" "Would I like to go and ingestionize some lunch?" If this is the price of fame, then 15 minutes is more than enough!

Which brings me to the major topic of my present communication. The FDA was brought into existence under the Federal Food Drugs and Cosmetics Act of 1938 with the best of intentions, namely to protect the public. It is now just one vehicle in a veritable traffic jam of federal agencies regulating virtually every aspect of American life. There is a certain irony in the fact, currently the focus of much political debate, that the United States—a nation founded on rugged individualism: a nation of pioneers—is probably more regulated than any country on earth. The United States certainly boasts more lawyers per capita than any country on earth, although many would argue that this is hardly anything to boast about.

The FDA regulates healthcare by controlling the marketing and labelling of drugs and medical devices by manufacturers: it is illegal for a company to market a drug or medical device in the United States without FDA approval. Investigational drugs and devices can only be distributed under the terms of an Investigational Drug/Device Exemption (IDE), which are rigorously controlled. It would not be strictly illegal for a physician to use a non-approved drug or device for patient treatment, although it is highly unlikely that he/she would ever manage to lay his/her hands on such an item. It would also be very difficult—if not impossible—to defend a lawsuit arising from the use of a drug or device that had not secured FDA approval: hardly worth the risk in a country with so many hungry, predatory lawyers. Moreover, third party payers—insurance companies, Medicare, etc.—would not reimburse the costs of such treatment, thereby making it simultaneously risky and unprofitable, effectively precluding its use.

While the marketing regulations for drugs and other therapeutic agents have little direct impact on laboratory haematology, the regulations pertaining to medical devices—a category that includes

---

Reprinted with permission of the author and Clinical and Laboratory Haematology, © 1995; 17(4):357–358. Edited from the original.

everything from prosthetic heart valves to diagnostic reagents—are critical. The Medical Device Amendments of 1976 and the Safe Medical Devices Act of 1990 established the FDA as the major agency responsible for the regulation of medical devices, requiring that manufacturers provide premarket notification of all medical devices to the FDA. Thus begins a lengthy, costly and often contentious procedure whereby devices are classified according to the scale of any damage that may potentially be inflicted on an unsuspecting populace. Briefly, Class I devices are those for which general controls—simple good manufacturing practices—are adequate to ensure safety and effectiveness. Class II devices are those for which Class I controls are insufficient, but for which safety and effectiveness can be assured by specific controls and requirements. Any device not falling into these categories is placed by default into Class III, requiring premarket approval. This means that the manufacturer must convince the FDA that the device is safe and effective before it can be sold. Class III status may well be the kiss of death for a new device, as the FDA is not exactly famous for its willingness to accept data at face value or to gloss over small and seemingly irrelevant details. Indeed, it is widely believed that obsessive compulsive personality disorder is an absolute requirement for prospective FDA employees.

Does the FDA contribute significantly to the public good? The same question could be asked of any regulatory organization. Does bureaucracy ever provide valid solutions to life's problems? In the case of the FDA, one would probably—on balance—answer "yes." But one would probably have to think twice or even three times before making up one's mind. Bureaucratic organizations such as the FDA move with all the speed and agility—not to mention the sensitivity—of a brontosaurus. Innovative products may thus be obsolescent by the time they pass through the regulatory system, assuming they are not trampled into oblivion by the process.

Having completionized my 1000 words it is time to terminationize my letter. Felicitationizations to all my readers.

SO YOU'VE JOINED A SOCIETY

Some members keep their society so strong,
While others join just to belong.
Some dig right in . . . some serve with pride;
Some go along just for the ride.
Some volunteer to do their share,
While some lie back and just don't care.
On meeting days some always show,
While there are those who never go.
Some always pay their dues ahead,
Some get behind for months instead.
Some do their best . . . some build . . . some make . . .
Some lag behind . . . some let things go;
Some never help their society grow.
Some drag . . . some pull . . . some don't . . . some do . . .
Consider . . . which one of these are you?

Reprinted with permission from Dental Assistant, © 1969; 38(10):24.

DEAR MR. BROWN

Russell L. Malone

Mr. Steven L. Brown
Chief Executive Officer
John Hancock Mutual Life Insurance
Boston, MA 02117

Dear Mr. Brown:

Mary Lou Blinkley and I are disappointed in you. Just in case you're not one of the 70,000 regular readers of *Asha*, let me explain that Mary Lou Blinkley is the girl whom Sister Mary Ellen put in charge of our fifth grade classroom when Sister had to leave. Mary Lou was very smart. Of course, all the kids hated her. I used to dream of the day that I'd become the class hero by showing Sister that I knew something, anything, that Mary Lou didn't.

That Friday morning started out just like every other day of school, with a prayer followed by "Please pass your homework to the person in front of you, and Mary Lou will collect it from the head of each row."

I was the head of my row, right in front of Sister's desk. I felt important in that power position, sometimes forgetting I was there only because Sister caught me talking to Roy Heyl during morning prayer.

"Children, we are going to have a quiz about names in American history. Who can tell me about Benjamin Franklin?"

Benjamin Franklin? Benjamin Franklin? Benjamin Franklin! That's the V & X on Oakmont Boulevard. V & X is what my sisters called it after they learned Roman numerals.

I raised my hand just as Sister said, "Mary Lou?"

"Benjamin Franklin discovered electricity by flying a kite in a rainstorm."

He did?

"Very good, Mary Lou. Russell, what were you going to say?"

"That's what I was going to say, Sister," I said, knowing that statement would cost me three Our Fathers and three Hail Marys when I went to confession.

"And who knows the name John Hancock?" asked Sister Mary Ellen smiling sweetly just like she had seen Ingrid Bergman do it in "The Bells of St. Mary's."

Nearly out of my seat with excitement, I waved my hand.

"Mary Lou . . ." Sister began.

Oh, damn, I thought and visions of three more Our Fathers and three Hail Marys crossed my mind.

". . . let's let Russell try first," continued Sister, not showing a lot of confidence, I noted.

"John Hancock is a life insurance company. They call it the rock!" I shouted, momentarily wondering if I had confused the rock with Alcatraz. I heard a titter come from Mary Lou's mouth as she waved her hand frantically.

"Mary Lou?"

"Sister, Russell is obviously thinking of Prudential," triumph oozing from every syllable. "You told us that John Hancock is the name of the man who signed the Declaration of Independence in big letters and said, 'I think King George can read that!'"

Knowing that Sister encouraged intelligent questions, I tried to recoup my near win. "Sister, which came first? John Hancock Insurance or John Hancock?"

I felt a sharp jab in my back as Ray Bluestone hissed, "Dummy."

"Well, Russell," said Sister-Ingrid-Bergman-smiling-sweetly, "both are highly respected names which have earned our admiration for their contribution to society."

Rubbing my back, I concluded that although not a clear victory, I had come off fairly well.

But, Mr. Brown, what do you think Sister Mary Ellen would say today? Sister has had a stroke in the intervening years and has trouble saying some words.

I hope she hasn't seen your commercial. You know, the one with the cute little girl who stutters. The one where you tell her to stop talking and use

---

Reprinted with permission of the author and ASHA, © 1992; 34(6/7):112. Edited from the original.

the word processor instead. That people won't laugh at her if she writes instead of talks. Boy, I wouldn't want to be there if you told Sister Mary Ellen to stop talking and write instead. Your palms would be stinging for days!

You wouldn't win any points by telling Sister that John Hancock's commercial won an award, either.

"Steven," Sister would ask, "just who gave you the award? People who have communication problems? Families of people who have communication problems? Professionals who help people become more effective communicators? The American Speech-Language-Hearing Association? The Stuttering Foundation of America? Is John Hancock as insensitive to other groups with special needs because they form only a small part of our population? I don't think so, Steven."

"But, Sister, most people who see it don't object."

"Steven, Steven, most people don't stutter!"

You won't get far, Mr. Brown, by telling Sister that your advertising agency said you have to stand behind the writer of your commercial, because he stutters. Sister used to tell us, "if you have a problem with your work, seek help, but if you do it wrong, you'll have to do it over again."

Oh, Sister can be tough when she feels that someone is sacrificing the good of others to satisfy his or her own selfish wants. "Money earned through the suffering of others is evil."

"But, Sister, what if we didn't know it was wrong?"

"Then it is a smaller sin, but you have to make it right." Sister had a saying to cover just about every wrong doing.

You'd also have to tell Sister that your advertising agency said it was a "closed matter," and that John Hancock intends to continue running this commercial, and "we'll just have to agree to disagree."

I wouldn't want to be in your shoes, Mr. Brown, if Sister hears about this. I won't tell Sister, Mr. Brown, and I won't urge our members to write to you, but you know Mary Lou Blinkley. She tells on everyone!

Sincerely,

Russ Malone

PHARMACY'S NEW (STARRING) ROLE

Doug Bennett, RPh

Now that the box office blitz of big-budget holiday movies is history, I am left with a box of stale popcorn and a question: Where are Hollywood's pharmacy heroes?

Why is it that we who wield the silver spatulas have yet to be featured on the silver screen? Granted, we've had more than our 15 minutes of cinematic fame. But I for one don't particularly enjoy being portrayed as a gap-toothed yokel whose sole professional purpose is to chase hormonally haunted teenagers away from the condom counter.

It's time to lose the stereotype. After all, does it take a quantum leap of logic to picture Cruise, Costner, or Clooney as dashing young pharmacists-in-charge facing danger around every corner drug store? It is really that hard to picture parents and their toy-crazed kids storming the local Toys R' Us for a shot at the latest Dash Druggist action figure? (Spatula sold separately.)

Unfortunately, the answers to these questions are painfully clear. Although pharmacy is "a life-saving profession," today's cinema buffs expect to see their on-screen heroes battle bombs, blades and bullets, not cut-throat contracts, fiendish formularies and villainous varicose veins.

With this in mind, I've developed a few pharmaco-cinematic plots of my own.

The producers of *The Pelican Placebo* proudly present . . . *A Time To Fill*. Tom Cruise stars as Dave Drylab, an ace pharmacy grad whose Pharm.D. degree and expertise in nuclear medicine have netted him an entry-level position at Wally's Drive-Thru Drug Mart and Deli.

One day, while billing third party scripts, Dave accidentally discovers U.P.A.C., the Universal Prior Authorization Code, which will allow *any* pharmacy to bill *any* HMO for *any* formulary-restricted drug and receive full payment, plus a generous consultation fee. Danger and suspense ensue as Dave attempts to e-mail the clandestine code to every pharmacy in the country, only to be trapped in a Website of intrigue as evil computer geeks transform his transmission into naughty pictures of Brad Pitt and his girlfriend. The film's advisory: "Warning: This movie may not be suitable for pre-pharmacy students."

If you liked *Voyage of the Drammed*, you'll love *Apothecary Harry and the Drug Reps of Doom*. Harrison Ford, star of such movies as *Indiana Jones and The Hollywood Cash-Cow*, swaps his trademark jacket and whip for a lab coat and a license-to-fill in this action-packed pharma-flick.

Harry, a rogue relief pharmacist and collector of pharmaceutical antiques, is in search of a rare pill tile upon which is inscribed the ultimate secret of operating a profitable pharmacy. Hounded by a band of HMO hoods led by the seductive Horizontal Floe, Harry at length obtains the coveted crumbling tile and deciphers the ancient Latin inscription which reads, "Never settle for less than AWP minus 10% plus a $2.50 filling fee you Doody Heads!" The advisory for this film: "Warning: Do not attempt to operate heavy machinery while watching this movie."

From the creators of the hit TV series comes a major motion picture . . . *The "Rx" Files*.

They call them "controlled drugs." But lately, they are out of control. Enter agents Sculder and Mully, a rag-tag duo of DEA washouts assigned the bizarre and "fuzzy" cases known collectively as the "Rx" files. (Cue: eerie music.) Summoned from their makeshift desks in the DEA's "dead letter" office (the room wherein thousands of defunct red

---

Reprinted with permission of the author and American Druggist, © 1998; 215(2):56–57. Edited from the original.

"C" stamps are stored), the agents are assigned to investigate strange reports of water-related disappearances of controlled drugs.

It seems that Valium is vanishing down toilet bowls. T-3s are being eaten by garbage disposals. And Vicodin is falling victim to the family washing machine. Here's a clip:

"This never happens with diuretics, only the controlled stuff," exclaims pharmacist Fred of Fill-4-Less Drugs, who is being grilled by the agents during his lunch break.

"Something very strange is going on here Mully," whispers Sculder.

"You mean the fact that certain drugs are exhibiting unusual hydrophilic tendencies?" asks Mully.

"Not exactly," Sculder continues. "Think about it. If in fact ol' Fred here really is a registered pharmacist . . . how come he gets a lunch break?"

Mully to Fred: "Freeze you alien scum!"

Warning: This movie contains gratuitous flashlight scenes.

I have many more ideas for movies that feature us, the real role models of society, risking our lives while counting by fives. However, the confines of space and good taste won't permit me to share them at this time. So if you happen to know any big-shot film producers, give me a call. Better still, have their people call my people. We'll meet. We'll schmooze. We'll do lunch. On second thought, better make that breakfast.

TODAY MIGHT BE DIFFERENT

There's something so satisfying just knowing that today will not be exactly like any work day that has gone before. It's almost enough to make you want to jump out of bed, greet the dawn, and rush off to work in a state of euphoria. Okay, so there aren't any awards given for showing up euphoric, but, still it could be a day for life-changing events. Today might be that one time when every obstacle is easily overcome and peace and harmony reign in the universe. Of course, it could also be a lot like yesterday, so try to prepare yourself for the unexpected.

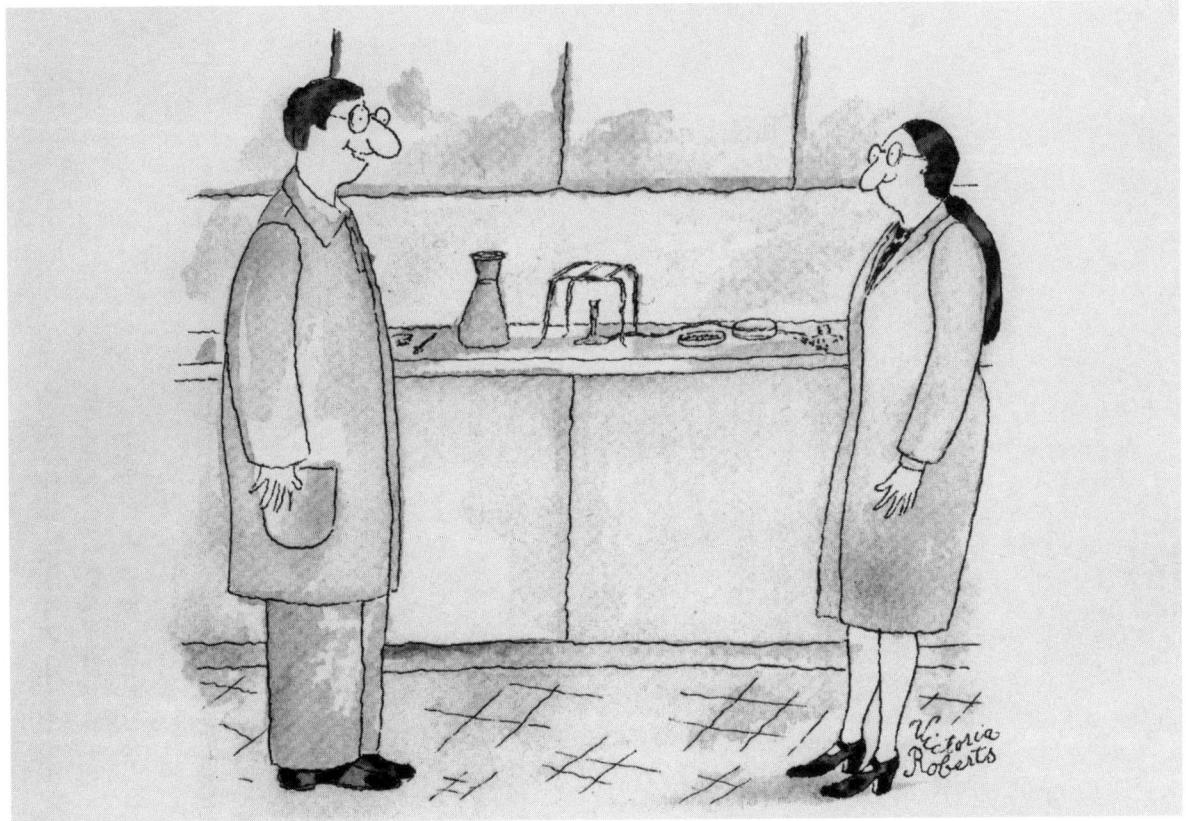

"We're in our lab coats. Now what?"

(© The New Yorker Collection 1998 Victoria Roberts from cartoonbank.com. All Rights Reserved.)

YOU SAY YOU WANT A RESOLUTION?

Jeff Lucia, NREMT-P

Jan. 1, 19-something-or-other. 7:59 a.m. I'm lying face-down on a bed, only dimly aware of my surroundings. Who am I? Where am I? *What* am I? Where was I last night, and what could I have done to deserve such a headache?

Fighting off the waves of nausea, I drag myself to the bathroom and hoist my face in front of the mirror. As the fluorescent light hums to life and begins to pummel my poor brain, some of the previous evening's festivities come back to me: Parties—several of 'em. Lots of drunk people breathing whiskey vapors in my face. A fight or two. Somebody puking on my shoes. A woman with . . . CHF and chest pain? And something about a nursing home and a CVA. . . .

"Lucia!" somebody's voice slams into my head. "You look like hell. And the rig's a mess . . . you're gonna clean it up before you take off, right?"

As holidays go, New Year's has never been particularly kind to me. It seems like I've worked enough shifts starting on Dec. 31 to make it through to Labor Day, and every one of them has been, to use a four-letter word, busy.

But even if you're lucky enough to get out of working New Year's Eve, you still have to deal with something almost as bad—thinking up New Year's resolutions. My list usually looks something like this:

1. Take down Christmas lights
2. Eat better, exercise more
3. Avoid working New Year's Eve next year

I don't know if your resolutions are any different, but in case you're having trouble coming up with your own, here are a few to get you started:

- **Resolve to become a better listener.** Let me ask you something: When was the last time you actually learned something while you were talking? Never? Didn't think so. Nature granted humans the remarkable ability to absorb knowledge, but for some reason, the process is short-circuited while the mouth is flapping. (Proof: If you've intubated any conscious patients, have you noticed how well they pay attention to you?) Even if you're Einstein, there's something you can learn from *every single person you meet*. Resolve to learn something new every day.

- **Resolve to be a better teacher.** It's far easier (and, OK, sometimes more fun) to let someone else flounder than to expend the energy to share your expertise. Remember when you were an EMS newbie? How you were an information black hole, absorbing every snippet of knowledge, helpful hint and trick of the trade you could? Well, chances are there's someone you work with who feels the same way. But a word to the wise: Nobody likes an overflowing fountain of knowledge, so speak and then shut up.

- **Resolve to trust others.** Nobody can start IVs, interpret rhythms, teach an EMT class, intubate, document, dispatch, drive or change the sheets on the stretcher better than you can. But that's no reason not to step back and let other people try. Besides, you might learn something. Trust your co-workers to run a shift or two without you, and spend the time with your family or pursuing some outside activity instead.

- **Live in the moment.** Whether you're in the middle of the most important call of your career or just relaxing with the important people in your life, stop for a second, take a deep breath, and remind yourself that *this moment right now* is your life. You're living it. Make the most of it.

- **Resolve to do something for yourself.** You know those TV interviews with people celebrating their 100th birthdays? How many have said that if they had their lives to live over again, the one thing they'd do is work more? There's a lot of value in those run-of-the-mill resolutions—eat better, exercise more, quit smoking—the things that help the most important person in your life: you.

So you say you want a resolution? Well, we all want to change the world . . . but let's start with ourselves. Now excuse me. I've got some Christmas lights to take down.

Reprinted with permission from JEMS: Journal of Emergency Medical Services, © 1995; 20(1):6.

BE A LEAN, MEAN, FILLING MACHINE

Doug Bennett, RPh

The practice of pharmacy makes many demands—on our time, our minds and our bodies. But these demands are not without benefits.

Time demands have made us excellent time managers, for he who survives counts quickly by fives. Mental stresses have honed our minds into finely tuned, fact-sorting machines, capable of translating hieroglyphic doctor doodles into drug names. And thanks to the physical demands associated with filling prescriptions, our bodies enjoy the muscle definition of the Pillsbury Doughboy.

The technical term is *flabbus pharmaceuticus*, a condition made worse by the infamous after-hours C.E. seminar dinner. "Uh . . . excuse me, folks. If you could just put down the prime rib and move away from the open bar, Dr. Bigbeamer will now discuss the etiology of coronary artery disease."

Many of you may have this condition and not even know it. Here are some tell-tale signs to watch for:

- Your apothecary globe is better proportioned than you are.
- You need a spatula extender to reach the pill tray.
- The Meridia rep says, "I never sample pharmacists . . . but in your case. . . ."
- A button pops off your smock, causing your entire staff to yell "incoming" and duck for cover.
- You drop a pill. Your tech says, "It's right there by your foot," and you have to ask, "Okay, so where's my foot?"

Well, what are you going to do about it? As I see it, you have three choices:

1. Join a gym where people with buns o'steel and washboard abs will make you feel like Jabba the Hut.

2. Buy your lab coats at Big Bertha's House O' Smocks.

3. Plug in to "Pharma Fitness," my powerful program of health-enhancing exercises that you can do during the course of your pill-filling day.

Just how effective is Pharma Fitness? Here's what some of your fellow pharmacists are saying:

"I was first introduced to Pharma Fitness by a close friend. After just one week, we were no longer on speaking terms."—Anna Filaxis, R.Ph., Humibid, LA.

"I gave Pharma Fitness a 90-day trial and before I knew it, three months had passed."—Al O'Purino, Benzac, WA.

So what are you waiting for? A prior authorization? Just do these workouts on a daily basis and in no time, customers and colleagues alike will be saying, "Gosh! There's something different about you. I know. You smell like a high school gym locker."

Are you ready? Okay. Just dial that radio to an up-tempo tune and . . . Hey, I said, UP-tempo! Like that Rolling Stones classic, "I Can't Get No Spatula Traction." Kenny G. and Yanni do not qualify. That's better. Okay, let's kick it!

Exercise No. 1

Fast-Mover Squats

Great for the thighs and for keeping the ol' gluteus maximus to a minimus. Begin by placing all your fast movers, i.e., Prozac, Xanax, Vicodin, (Hey, I'm in southern California, okay?) on the bottom shelves. This, instead of placing them conveniently in front of you where you can reach them with all the energy expenditure required to operate your TV remote. Reach for the drugs by bending at the knees, doing several repetitions throughout the day.

Then reach for that other fast mover, Motrin. You'll need it.

Exercise No. 2

Wrists of Steel

For this exercise, you will need to duct-tape a five-pound weight to the handle of your spatula. As you

Reprinted with permission of the author and American Druggist, © 1998; 215(8):54–55.

count out the pills or mix up those ointments, the extra weight resistance will strengthen your wrists and forearms. For maximum benefit, alternate hands. That is, if you can find a left-handed pill tray.

Exercise No. 3

Drug-Rep Dodges

Great for the pharmacists in stores frequented by reps bearing high-fat freebies. At the first sign of a pizza or pastry-packing rep, quickly duck behind the counter. The downside of this exercise is that you will also miss out on the other cool stuff the reps bring. Hey. Did I say downside?

Exercise No. 4

Jug Lugs

A great way to buff up the biceps and pecs. First replace all those puny pint-sized cough syrup bottles with glass gallon jugs. When a cough syrup script comes in, take a deep breath and pour the desired liquid from the jug using the scientific method known as "Jed Clampett's homemade moonshine pouring technique." Exhale completely and wipe your brow thoroughly. Then wipe up all the spilled syrup, but watch your language in front of the pediatric suspensions.

Exercise No. 5

Fatigue Mat Treadmill

Pick a low-traffic area of your anti-fatigue mat and pour out 50 to 100 Tessalons. You will now discover that you can walk briskly upon the "Tessalon-treated" mat in true treadmill fashion. This is good for your cardiovascular system but bad for the Tessalons (and your bottom line), as they cannot be used in any future prescriptions.

Note: To maximize heart rate during this exercise, review your third-party contracts, paying particular attention to reimbursement rates.

So there you have it. A comprehensive exercise routine for the busy pharmacist. I challenge you to try it for just 30 days—preferably in a row. Soon you'll be a lean mean filling machine. You'll also be collecting Worker's Comp.

Oh, and one more thing. Be sure to watch for my upcoming Pharma Fitness video, "Sweatin' To The Formularies."

SUMMER ADVICE:

More Than Just Sunscreen
Montgomery Vickers, OD

By now everyone has heard that strange song/poem/commencement speech that drones on about suntan lotion or whatever. I never get that far, because the instant it comes on, I immediately switch the station in pursuit of Pink Floyd or Shania Twain.

When this piece of work hit the Internet, the scuttlebutt was that it was secretly authored by Kurt Vonnegut, Jr. who, as every optometrist worth a sample of latanoprost knows, introduced the world to our famous colleague, Billy Pilgrim, O.D., in *Slaughterhouse Five*. And, since I found out this song/poem/commencement speech was a hoax, I refuse to listen. Besides, I only read or listen to eye doctors. OK, I only read and listen to myself. At least I admit it.

Reprinted from Review of Optometry, © 1999; 136(8):23, with permission of the author.

So I decided I could do better. Funny thing about egos. I hope this helps refocus you oldies and inspires—as it should—you kids. So here it is, MY "UV-Blocking Lenses," not by Kurt Vonnegut, Jr.

Wear UV-blocking lenses. After all, they couldn't hurt and you only have one set of eyes. And by the way, you should be nice to your Mom and Dad. They do have Medicare, and that's more than you'll ever have. Maybe you can co-manage their cataracts, unless you're chicken.

Always keep 20 ones, 10 tens and 10 fives in the cash box. The one day you don't will be the day you forget your wallet. Just try to find enough change in the seats of your minivan to upsize your burger!

Speak kindly to your sales reps. They have a hard job trying to control their impulses to wrap their fingers around your scrawny neck and choke you until you squeak like the Mayor of Munchkinland. Yes, they make good money, but most of it goes for Kava Kava.

Tell your receptionist you love her. No, don't tell her that. She'll slap you with a sexual harassment suit. Instead tell her you think her dress is pretty. No, that's grounds for a suit, too. Try this: Tell her you like her hair. No . . . just tell her you need Mrs. Smith's chart.

Be patient with new presbyopes. When someone fusses about her new bifocals, try to understand when she says, "I can't see," instead of calling 911 to call her bluff because she just said she was blind. She may have meant something else.

Take 10 percent of every dollar you bring in and put it in the "I forgot your birthday and/or anniversary fund." Don't argue. Just do.

Take your teen-ager's face into your hands, look him in the eyes and say, "You can be anything you want in the whole world . . . except a millionaire in one year, if you follow the psychic's advice." Also, tell him that the key to good communication with a parent is to shut the hell up during the ball game.

Open your mind to new things, unless they have anything to do with having to buy a contact lens bank.

Always make friends. When you leave a room, make certain that those left behind say something nice, and not something like, "Optometrists sure do smell funny."

Make plans. Set goals. It's not enough to say, "I need a margarita." You must buy a lime and some salt.

Walk into your optical. My God, how many little, round, preppy frames must you have? Buy something gaudy and charge a lot for it.

Stop whining about every little thing. Your life is wonderful. It could be worse. You could have a 16-year-old kid with a Mensa IQ. Thank the Lord that you don't have to debate Sherlock Freakin' Geraldo F. Lee Baily Vickers about what time the 11 o'clock curfew is.

Give yourself a break. You're not perfect. Only your spouse is perfect. At least MINE is.

Hold someone in esteem. Respect a peer, a colleague. Choose a mentor. Learn all you can. Then crush 'em like a gnat and find a new one.

If you're gonna cuss, then cuss with abandon. If you're not gonna cuss, then respect those who can.

Oh, and don't forget . . . use those UV-blocking lenses, but don't presume for a second that they'll prevent cataracts in an 80-year-old. She already has 'em. It's just your slit lamp that sucks.

Kurt would be proud.

HELLO MUDDA, HELLO FADDA

...A Letter From Camp PT

Peter Kovacek, MS, PT

Monday

Here I am at Camp Physical Therapy. It has been six months since I graduated and I'm really glad I came here. It is a wonderful place. All the time and energy and money we put into preparing me to come to camp really was worth it. The patients are great, I really seem to be making a difference with them, I just wish I had more time to spend with them.

The gang here is really great too. Even Maria, the boss, is pretty cool. I can talk to her almost any time I want. She sure seems to have a tough job, though. She keeps telling us about something changing that will really affect us a lot. But then she tells us that we are all working hard and getting along well—so "keep up the good work." I am so glad that she is satisfied with the way we do things.

I am pretty satisfied, too. I get to spend time with each of my patients every time they come in for therapy. That is really important, 'cuz you know that the only way patients get better is when I treat them—the more the better. I was worried when I graduated from PT school that I would not get to treat the way I wanted to. But here at Camp Physical Therapy, I decide what I will do. I'm a professional.

Today was a really, really good day. I am treating Mr. Jones for a stroke and he is coming along very well. I got to spend more than an hour of time with him today. We were working on his walking and he is really improving. I have really enjoyed the five months that we've been working together. Mr. Jones was one of my first patients here at Camp. I hope I treat him forever.

Maria is glad to see Mr. Jones doing so well. She even wants me to think about the time when he won't need therapy any more. That will probably be a long time. Maria also mentioned something about me seeing more patients because of the waiting list, but I told her that I was going to give Mr. Jones and all my patients the best care possible. So, I want to be sure to have enough time to work with them. Besides, the patients on the waiting list are not my problem. Why should Mr. Jones suffer just because a bunch of other people are waiting? It would be unethical for me to change my treatment for Mr. Jones just because of the waiting list. Wouldn't it?

Tuesday

I really like Maria. She came to me again and we had a lovely chat. But she sure seems tense and overworked. Her boss, Fred, seems like a real tough guy to deal with. He is not like the rest of us. Maria told me that Fred is pushing her to change things and try to get more patients. I told Maria to stick to her guns and stand up to Fred. She asked for my help and I told her that she could count on me to support her.

Wednesday

Apparently, Maria spoke to most of the gang here at Camp. Everybody is real concerned about her. We had a meeting and decided that Fred is too mean to Maria. We decided to write him a letter and tell him to leave Maria alone. We are all very happy here at Camp Physical Therapy. We don't want things here to change. The patients also like it here. Some of my patients have gone to other therapy camps and they always tell me bad things about those places. We told Fred that we don't want this camp to turn into one of those places where all they do is treat lots of patients. It is different here. We care about our patients and get to spend as much time with them as we want. We are all glad that we don't have to worry about all that managed

ADVANCE for Physical Therapists, © 1998; 9(10):6. This article has been reprinted with permission from ADVANCE Newsmagazines.

care and reimbursement stuff. All we have to do is treat our own patients well and every two weeks we get paid.

Thursday

Maria was off today. She called in sick. I am glad she took the time off, she didn't look good yesterday. Way over tired. I think she misses treating patients. I know I would. We all got a note today that said Fred wanted to meet with us at lunch on Friday. I guess he got our letter. Good! I knew we could work this out. It worked just like in the books that we read in school. When people communicate, it all works out. Fred just needed to understand the way things work here in physical therapy. We all know that he is not one of us, so we were glad to set him straight.

Friday

So, Mom and Dad, how are you? Have I told you recently how much I love you? Today was not a good day. Fred came to that meeting I told you about. He told us that Maria won't be our boss anymore. Fred said that camp was just not making enough money to continue with Maria in charge. He also said that we were all going to have to see more patients every day. He said we weren't performing at the level of most of our competitors so there will probably be a hiring freeze and maybe even some staff reductions. I am the newest person at Camp, so I am sure I will get fired. If only Fred understood physical therapy better. Camp just isn't as much fun as it is supposed to be anymore.

CAMP PT IS LOOKING BETTER

Dan Dandy, PT

The letter home from 'Camp PT' tells of a change of heart for the newest camper

Saturday

Mom and Dad: I was feeling down last night so I went for a walk. Along the way, I met one of the older patients here at the camp. He asked why I was so glum.

I explained that camp had changed and that I don't think camp PT is right for me any more. I told him that my only desire is to help the ill or injured, to help people who need me. Instead, I told him, I find myself with constraints I never learned about in school nor had during my early years at the camp. He patiently listened to me as I lamented about insurance companies and productivity, mergers and managed care. I confessed that I was planning to pack my bags and find a different kind of camp.

Expecting sympathy, I was surprised by his response. He said:

"I've heard these complaints before. I have watched as many bright, caring and creative therapists have come to camp only to leave disgruntled. Such a waste of schooling, knowledge and potential. I hear your claim of noble aspiration and benevolent ideals. Unfortunately, it seems you have the misconception that because you have 'honorable' intentions, the road to their implementation should be smooth and the journey painless.

"Your degree was an admission ticket to a participant not a spectator event.

"If you truly want to help those of us who are ill or injured, why are you leaving? Never before have patients needed therapists with those qualities you aspire to as they do now. Never before has

ADVANCE for Physical Therapists, © 1998; 9(13):82. This article has been reprinted with permission from ADVANCE Newsmagazines.

there been an opportunity to make a difference in our lives and in the direction of your profession. Never before have patients needed therapists as they do now.

"Imagine you had a loved one receiving your care. Would you be packing your bags? Of course not. You would be using your creativity and expertise as well as knowledge of the health care system in the most effective and efficient manner you could. You would be looking for ways to maximize your treatments while seeking long-term solutions to the changes you feel compromise the quality of PT."

Sunday

Mom and Dad: I think I might be staying at this camp for awhile. I've been thinking, maybe I can make a difference at camp after all.

AN ODE TO CALL TECHNOLOGISTS

Oh the woes and the trials of the call tech at night,
When the ring of the phone brings on such a great fright

Like Pavlov's good dog, we're conditioned it's true
At the sound of the bell, we know just what to do

We stumble from bed with a quite foggy brain,
And growl about the hour, which seems so insane

For while civilized people are home in their beds,
We're x-raying drunks with cuts on their heads

Or perhaps it's a chest that's been called a code blue,
Or TMJ tomos, or a C.T. scan too

But whatever the request, it's always called STAT,
Which keeps us poor techs from getting too fat

The wait by the processor seems endless you know,
Is the film dark enough, did your markers all show?

When the patients keep coming and there's no end in sight,
You get that horrible feeling that you're here for the night

It might help you to think of the money you're making,
Try to forget all those taxes Uncle Sam will be taking

Because the money is trivial in comparison to
The knowledge you've gained, when at last you are through

For, who else but a call tech, can rise from the deep,
And take quality x-rays when they're still half asleep?

Written in the middle of the night by an anonymous call tech.

Reprinted with permission from Radiologic Technology, © 1988; 59(4):349.

BATHROOM HUMOR

Kathy Sitzman, BSN, RN

As a home care nurse working in what my employer refers to as an "outlying area," I cover a vast territory of both rural and urban settings. Due to a genetically predetermined condition called Miniature Bladder Syndrome, I have toiled to develop an intricate knowledge of public restrooms in my region. I thrill with the discovery of an easily accessible, nonrepulsive restroom.

Last week, I drove 60 miles to the main office for meetings. Road construction along the way led to frequent traffic backups. To pass away the time, I sang along with an oldies tape and sipped a rather large cup of iced tea. It would be an understatement to describe my condition as desperate as I approached the exit ramp at snail speed. Because I didn't see any restrooms between the exit and the office, I opted for the sure thing and sped toward the office amidst squealing tires and flying bags and clipboards.

Following a spectacular side-sliding entry into the parking lot, I bolted through the back door and ran straight for the ladies room. "I'll be with you in a minute," I called over my shoulder. The nurses I passed nodded knowingly in my direction.

After the meeting, I asked for advice on restrooms in the area. A crowd gathered and enthusiastically shared their data.

"Zeke's Gas-A-Teria is pretty clean but hard to find," said one.

"Lumpy's Fuel Emporium is on the main drag and has three stalls and a water fountain, but Old Lumpy gets mad if you use the john and don't buy gas," added another.

Another coworker commented, "Gloria's Gas-O-Rama is clean and right behind Dwayne's Donuts on First Street. Parking is a problem in the morning because of all the squad cars parked in front of the donut shop."

I made a mental note of these and other suggestions before hurrying away to another meeting. While at the meeting, I chuckled at the thought of creating a public restroom resource list. How useful this list would be to those of us who spend time on the road. Of course it would require a rating system. As the meeting droned on, the idea took root and grew.

Restroom Rating System
* **Untidy Bowl:**
   Potential health hazard; use only in an emergency.
** **The Uninvited Guest Rest:**
   Toilet paper and soap usually available.
*** **The Restroomer:**
   Toilet paper and soap available; bug free; heated in winter.
**** **The Royale Flush:**
   Includes all amenities featured in Restroomer; regular emptying of trash receptacles; hot running water; functional stall latches; spiffy décor.

A computer database listing all regional restrooms would follow. After that, a Web page (updated weekly) and a 24-hour hotline referred to as the Throne Phone.

What can I say? It was a long meeting and my imagination took over. However, if a hotline *were* available, I'd have the number programmed into my cellular phone's speed dial.

Reprinted with permission from Home Healthcare Nurse, © 1998; 16(11):786.

YOUR GUIDE TO FEIGNING CIVILITY

Barbara M. Morris, RPh

Excuse me, is it just me? Is anyone else tired of being interrupted with a demanding "excuse me" at the most inappropriate times? It doesn't matter what you are doing—whether on the phone, in a personal conversation, concentrating on your work—some inconsiderate klutz who can't wait until you finish what you are doing will butt in with "excuse me." And woe be unto you if you ignore the intruder or take offense at the interference.

"Excuse me" is now the politically correct and socially acceptable means to engage in a feigned civility that used to be considered plain old-fashioned rudeness.

The other day I was on the phone in the pharmacy taking a prescription from a doctor. As he was giving lengthy and somewhat complicated instructions to be placed on the label, I heard a Voice at the counter.

"Excuse me?" said the Voice. It had a demanding edge to it, but that's okay; the Voice did utter the words "excuse me."

Choosing to stay focused on what the doctor was saying I ignored the Voice—but not for long. Two seconds later I heard it again.

"Ex-cuse me?" the Voice persisted, louder and more strident. But again, no offense taken; the Voice did intone the sacred words "excuse me."

At about this time the doctor had changed his mind about how he wanted the patient to take the medicine. Trying to listen to him and hush the Voice at the same time, I made eye contact with the Voice and put up my hand to indicate he had been heard. That was a mistake because the Voice took it as permission to be even more impatient.

"EX-CUSE ME," persisted the agitated Voice. "I just want to know where you keep your lice shampoo!" Although he did use the magic words, I still felt irritated. But I asked the doctor if he would excuse me for a moment. I then placed my hand over the phone mouthpiece and politely said to the Voice, "Excuse me, I'm on the phone. I'll help you as soon as I can." I then took the phone to a corner where I concluded my conversation with the doctor.

The Voice remained stationed at the counter, poised to do battle.

"Lady, you are (an unmentionable word that begins with 'B'). All I want to know is where you keep your lice shampoo." (Excuse me, dear reader, let me get your perspective about this. I'd say that calling me an uncouth name was not okay because he did not preface it with 'excuse me.' Do you agree with me? Am I right about that? I am right? Thank you.)

"Excuse me?" I replied with perfect patience, "lice shampoo is in aisle five." He left and I assumed I had seen the last of him, but he was back faster than a lice infestation can shut down a preschool.

"I don't see it. Get somebody to help me find it," he demanded.

I called for help—promptly. "We need customer service for lice shampoo in aisle five" I announced over the loudspeaker. Help did not arrive fast enough and wanting to provide excellent customer service, I called again. "Customer needs help with lice in aisle five!"

"You're rude. You are trying to embarrass me," the Voice snarled. "I'm going to report you to the manager."

Moi? Rude? Okay, I admit I failed to preface my announcement with "excuse me" Mea culpa! Mea maxima culpa! I quickly reconsidered my social sin of omission and began a thoughtful response with the proper penitential words.

"Excuse me," I said, oozing with compassion, "I'm just trying to be helpful, to anticipate all possible needs." Indulging in a little self-puffery I added with undisguised pride, "I won an award for providing excellent customer service." I added, "I'm sure the manager will be here soon and you can report me and you have a nice day." I reveled in the

Reprinted with permission of the author and American Druggist, © 1999; 216(1):52–53.

knowledge that the Voice was not going to have a nice day until he got his lice shampoo.

Two minutes later the manager appeared. The Voice chewed him out for making him wait and complained about my demeanor. After the Voice left with his lice shampoo, the manager called me aside.

"Excuse me, Barbara, the customer said you were nasty. What's going on?"

"Excuse me, he didn't tell me I was nasty—just rude."

"So why were you rude?"

"Excuse me, I wasn't rude."

"Excuse me, Madam Pharmacist," the manager curtly countered, "you must have been rude or he wouldn't have complained." (The customer is never wrong.) After a little more no-win repartee the manager left, scratching his head. Wanting to show him how helpful I can be, I quickly called out to him, "Lice shampoo is in aisle five."

The last I saw of the manager that day he was headed in the direction of aisle five. Could it be? Had I correctly anticipated an unspoken need? Had I once again justified my customer service award?

There is a two-part moral here.

Part One: Any behavior is acceptable as long as it is prefaced with "excuse me." (Even if a robber sticks a gun in your ribs and demands all your Vicodin—No generics, please!—if s/he prefaces "This is a stickup" with "excuse me"—s/he has what passes for good manners these days and that must be respected.)

Part Two: No matter what the customer wants, always offer the location of lice shampoo as well. Even if it doesn't earn you a customer service award, you may make a sale. Your boss might appreciate your keen powers to discern his unspoken needs as well. Then again, he might not. Avoid using the store intercom system to let him know that the lice shampoo is in aisle five.

And just in case you missed the message, be sure to preface everything you say with "excuse me." It's the nineties way to win friends and influence people.

A IS FOR AARDVARK . . .

Daniel Merton

For a time, Dr. Barry Goldberg and I provided ultrasound services to the Philadelphia Zoo. The animal keepers there had an aardvark that was pregnant. This particular aardvark had carried several times before but, unfortunately, never delivered a viable newborn. The keepers were interested to know how far along was the gestation. We had performed ultrasound studies on several of her prior pregnancies to the point where they were beginning to put together some biometric data to enable the dating of aardvark gestations.

I had to do a scan on this pig-like, plump beast and the only place she would allow us to lay her down without too much fuss was deep inside her "den," a dimly lit pseudo-cave with a plexiglass viewing window for the public. So, in I go toting along the ADR scanner and a 3.5-mHz transducer. (Dr. Goldberg observed through the window. Surprised?)

It was winter in the Northeast and I vividly recall that I had on a favorite all-wool sweater. It got pretty hot and very stinky being in a heated den designed for a single aardvark along with the ultrasound machine, Mrs. Aardvark, and her closest animal handler (i.e., "support human") to help comfort her during the sonogram. I did our usual "level II scan" (we don't do level I scans at Thomas Jefferson) and it was quite interesting. The fetal head was, as you might guess, elongated and had a very prominent snout. In many ways, it was similar

Reprinted with permission from Journal of Diagnostic Medical Sonography, © 1999; 15(1):32.

to a scan on a human—we mammalians being as alike as we are.

I'll never forget the faces of the few spectators through the viewing windows as they observed an obstetric sonogram being performed on an aardvark! I'll also never forget that nice, warm, wool sweater that I had to discard because, regardless of how many times we (okay, my wife!) tried, we could never completely eliminate the smell of the pregnant aardvark.

As I recall, that particular pregnancy did go to term and she delivered a healthy baby aardvark. I don't remember whether mom wanted to know the gender of the baby or whether it mattered to her at all. I believe the comment made was "as long as it's healthy . . ." I also do not recall whether it was a boy or girl. The memories at the zoo will last a lifetime, but I wish I still had that sweater.

Other memorable events in my career include:

1. The infertility patient who wanted me to be her artificial insemination donor because she thought I had "the most perfect nose." I declined. Thanks anyway.

2. The obviously native-Italian woman who, after I completed an abdominal scan on her elderly husband, gratefully urged me to visit her apparel store for a free package of underwear. "Youse a-gotta come-a our store in-a South Philly . . ." She even asked me my size and whether I used boxers or briefs! I declined that one, too.

FAST! WARM! FUZZY! EMERGENCY!

David Wolman, PA-C

Stream of consciousness is what Freud viewed as a person's thoughts verbalized as uninhibitedly as possible. Here is the stream of my consciousness during a shift in the ED where I am employed. Freud needed a hundred volumes to explain this; I'll be brief. And forgive my honesty. It comes with the Stream.

Preparations Are Made

I am carrying two Chef Boyardee low-fat, low-cholesterol beef ravioli microwave meals, a product that recently received preliminary approval from the FDA as edible food. The packages are about the size of a hockey puck—truly lifesavers, with a 90-second microwave time. They enable me to spend only 15 minutes eating two meals during my 12-hour shift.

I have just logged in today's hours in the physicians' lounge. There are two books: one in which physicians record academic time, administrative time, on-call, CME, meetings, and vacation; the other is for PAs to record their work hours.

I have donned my white coat over blue scrubs and filled the pockets with essential clinical gizmos collected over the years. With accoutrements, the coat weighs 80 pounds, which keeps me from floating with joy at the thought of working windowless for 12 hours, not including a 45-minute commute, on the most beautiful day of the year.

No Sooner Do I Enter

A nurse approaches me. He has just graduated and he is very bubbly. He tells me that an 18-year-old male is in the waiting room. The patient had a 90% pulse ox on arrival but don't worry, the nurse reassures me, no wheezes now!

This patient has been here before, and ended up on a ventilator. His father, by the way, is an oncologist.

Reprinted with permission from Journal of the American Academy of Physician Assistants, © 1997; 10(12):75–76, 78–79.

Oh, the nurse concludes, and he takes asthma medicine. The triage nurses have given the patient one nebulizer treatment out front. There are 20 patients ahead of him whose acuity ranges from plantar warts to blepharitis.

My brain, which hasn't yet been fed even a single helping of Chef Boyardee ambrosia, goes into high gear (picture a Hyundai with 200,000 miles): Low pulse ox. Asthma. No wheezes. Father is a doctor. . . . The longer I work in the ED, the more I think in simple terms. Because things can go down hill VERY SIMPLY.

My face drains of blood. I tell the nurse to put the patient in a room immediately. He asks me if it is OK to take the patient out of turn just because his father is a doctor. No, it is not okay to do this because his father is a doctor, I say. It is OK to do this because people who aren't breathing take preference.

The nurse is no longer smiling or bubbly. He retrieves the patient, puts him in Room 4, and informs me that he will be writing me up for, uh, something.

I don't greet the parents of the asthmatic boy—not because I am rude but because I can't help but notice that their son is using every accessory muscle I have ever seen and then some to breathe. His nostrils flare and he looks, well, a touch dusky. I inform my supervising physician that, without having examined the boy completely, my best judgment is that he is in imminent danger of respiratory failure despite a rejuvenating 2 hours in the waiting room.

Various orders are given. We start a nebulizer treatment but the nurse cannot find Atrovent to add to the albuterol because we are in the Fast Track area; emergency airway meds are in the core ED. We start an IV. We'd like to give steroids, but they are on back order from L.L. Bean. The nurse runs back and forth from the core, which is full, to our Fast Track, like someone in a nutty relay race on an old TV show.

Dad the oncologist is ominously silent but Mom, who reports that the boy was intubated previously in the ED, goes ballistic. Why would a mother be so emotional? I mean, her kid is going to need to be tubed any minute; they've been delayed for 2 hours; he is in the wrong part of the ED; and my supervising physician and I are missing only Curly to present a darn good imitation of the Three Stooges. Talk about overreaction!

We decide to move the patient to the core immediately. If they don't have room, that's their problem. (Actually, there are plenty of rooms—just not enough nurses to open them. We've played this game before.)

We'd like an oxygen bottle to move the patient. I run around looking for one. None in Fast Track. None in the core. The patient now does an excellent job of breathing with toe muscles. Finally, I find a bottle on a wheelchair out front. The patient in the chair has been waiting to have his emergent impacted cerumen cared for, so I shake off the thought that depriving him of oxygen will be brought up at the next QI meeting.

All we need now is an IV pole. None can be found. I grab the IV bag in my teeth, enhancing my professional demeanor, and away we go!

Now we're on a run with the stretcher at about 40 mph, the physician pushing and me steering. Mom swats me with her pocketbook to let off steam. The smacks are invigorating, a wonderfully refreshing beginning to my shift.

We arrive in the core. In seconds the patient is tubed. All is well. I'm grateful Dad is a doctor, because he knows how bad care can be. A normal person would have been shocked. (Mom? She called me later to apologize for the whacks and to thank me for quick action.) Only 15 minutes gone by, but I feel like I've lived through a millennium.

Can't Get Much Worse. Right?

That's my question as I sip lukewarm decaf tea. But then a colleague hands me an envelope. In it is a graph—one of those new graphs that people who go to school for medical administration learn how to construct. The note attached says that, according to the graph, which cannot lie, I'm not seeing the appropriate number of patients quickly enough.

Hey, 15 minutes for respiratory arrest! How fast do they want me to work? Oh I get it. They're talking about *real* Fast Track patients—suture removals, lacerations, abrasions, sprains, things you can really move quickly—meaning in 5 minutes. Problem is that half the time when I pick up a chart in Fast Track it's overflow from the core, meaning a very sick patient who fell through the triage sieve.

So this graph—created by someone who never sets foot in the ED for fear of stepping in something disgusting—this graph is irrelevant to what I do. This is the New World of Medicine. Things are measured and made more efficient and cost-effective.

The only problem is that the things that are measured and made more efficient and cost-effective are not the things people do in an ED.

Another Chart, Another Medical Precedent

Migraine. Patient states she is allergic to just about every OTC and Rx analgesic approved for use in this country (see Table 1). Prophylactic meds don't work. Only Demerol works. Patient has listed an out-of-state physician.

I enter the room. The lights are out and the patient, in dark glasses, sprawls across the stretcher. No movement. I introduce myself quietly. She does not answer. Thankfully, however, she is accompanied by Tattoo-Man, self-made migraine expert, who will interpret her pain for her. Usually, he says, she gets 150 mg Demerol IM and 100 Percocets to go. I examine the migraineur and retire to my office.

I admit to a disagreement with Administration on this type of patient. Administration thinks that patient satisfaction is more important than the World Bank, that our job is to give the patient what she wants despite our medical judgment, give it to her fast, and be warm and fuzzy about it. My feeling is, yes, it is expedient to give the Demerol, but if the patient suffers from drug addiction, not headache, it is proper medicine to treat the real problem.

I call the patient's physician, dialing a number supplied by Tattoo-Man, but there's no listing for this doctor. Does this physician, in fact, exist? Maybe in Paraguay, but not the United States.

Uh-oh. My 15-minute turnaround time is about up. I feel like Lucille Ball trying to keep up with the conveyer belt of candy. (Nickelodeon reruns are my frame of reference).

I explain that narcotics may only create rebound headaches—about as easy as explaining that a virus does not respond to antibiotics. Tattoo-Man fingers the Bowie knife on his belt; the patient under the sheet moans Chopin's Funeral March.

I confer with my supervising physician du jour (he's standing in for the regular Fast Track doc, who is at Disney World). He thinks Demerol is short and sweet. I must obey. Sure, I could raise a stink, but what would I get out of it? Be named designated complainer? We are a dependent profession.

Unprecedented History of Analgesic Failure in a Migraine Patient

Efficacy	Agent or Class
Ineffective*	β-Blockers
	Calcium-channel blockers
	Compazine
	Darvocet
	DHE
	Imitrex
	Motrin
	Phenergan
	Reglan
	Stadol
	Thorazine
	Toradol
	Tylenol
	Ultram
Effective*	Demerol

* Source: Tattoo-Man (personal communication, 1997).

Nurses can refuse to perform orders contrary to their scope of practice; PAs cannot. We're physician extenders, not physician pretenders. There, I've said it and I feel better.

I order the Demerol. In the meantime, I schedule 20 PAs and the medical residents for moonlighting shifts over the next 3 months. I sketch out three articles for publication and give the PA student a quick summary of lupus. I long for my second Chef Boyardee, but it's too early. With gourmet food, you have to pace yourself.

All Along the Vertebrae

Next patient has had back pain for 10 years. I must cure it in 15 minutes. He tells me he has a herniated disc at L4–S1. Or is it L6–S12? He can't remember, but he's sure something is wrong with his L's and S's. I ask the obvious: Who is taking care of his back problem? Why is he *here* now? He tells me he is in pain, it's Saturday and his physician is not available, and he is allergic to everything except— hold on, don't tell me—Demerol! Should I consult my supervising physician? Or jump ahead to the obvious?

This time I get the patient's physician on the telephone. I am relieved to find that the doctor is real, and a very nice guy, too. He tells me the patient has a substance abuse problem related to Vietnam (even though he never was there), his wife (the patient's wife), job stress (he is unemployed), and fibromyalgia, chronic fatigue syndrome, and temporomandibular joint dysfunction (all diagnosed by a chiropractor). He tells me to just give the Demerol and to ask the patient to see him on Monday.

I tell the nurse to hook up a large-gauge copper pipe to a huge vat of Demerol and start the IV.

Homeward Unbound

Eleven hours later, and I have taken care of fractured ankles, ingrown toenails, 12 children's fevers that would have responded nicely to Tylenol or Motrin had their parents given it, migraines, muscle aches, abrasions, burns, and a boxer's fracture in a guy who punched his refrigerator. I have stapled scalp lacerations, sutured another 10 or so, made splints for sprains and fractures (orthopods will only come in for patients who carry an extremity in a box), removed foreign bodies from eyes with a slit lamp and a needle, removed three foreign bodies from noses and two from other orifices, including a moth from an ear canal, called in dental consults on broken teeth and abscesses, treated toothaches with my Motrin-Tylenol with Codeine-Penicillin triad, x-rayed a penny in a baby's tummy, diagnosed external hemorrhoids and referred the patient to surgical clinic, diagnosed two cases of plantar fasciitis, given out 18 work excuses, written several thousand Motrin scrips (I exaggerate), and, yes, indulged in Chef Boyardee.

Buried in the mundane, I discovered meningitis, appendicitis, new-onset diabetes, cardiomyopathy in a 30-year-old whose only complaint was a cough that wouldn't quit, and active TB that presented as a cyst on the neck.

As I think about this on my way home, I notice flashing lights behind me. The state trooper recognizes me from the ED.

"Hey, *doc*, you don't have a license to speed."

I tell him he's absolutely right; I *don't* tell him that I am rushing home to catch a rerun of "ER." The work looks like so much fun there. Of course, if you add up commercial breaks and divide by the number of cases seen on an average episode—these people should be fired! Their graphs are terrible.

But the ratings are good. And that's what counts.

LAWS OF THE O.R.

March L. Warn, RN, CNOR

1. All equipment works until the moment it is needed.

2. The length of the line at the hospital cafeteria is directly proportionate to the number of cases on the surgery schedule.

3. Skinny people never need total joint replacements.

4. The number of items you will need to leave the room for during the surgical procedure is directly proportionate to the distance to the supply room.

5. Laundry services will always find the 99 cent Bic lighter you left in the pocket of your scrub clothes, but will never find the new Rolex watch in there with it.

6. Payroll will only lose your time card for the pay period preceding the due date of your car/mortgage payment.

7. The only instrument you will drop during a surgical procedure is the one for which there is no back-up.

8. Surgeons will be consistent in their routines unless you are training a new employee.

9. The surgeon who has not worked in your OR for the last fifteen years will call to schedule a case the day after you throw out all his preference cards.

10. Any major piece of equipment will be on the opposite side of the room from where the surgeon wants it.

11. Surgeons will consistently use a special charge item unless it is opened before they ask for it.

12. Patients who are the most concerned about the cosmetic results of their surgeries are the least likely to suffer from a large, ugly scar.

13. Spinal anesthetics work most consistently on the rectal sphincter.

14. Any weather disturbance (blizzard, tornado, flood, etc.) of sufficient magnitude to prevent half of the staff from getting to work will not be severe enough to prevent any of the same day surgery patients from getting to the hospital.

15. The chances of any outpatient canceling his or her surgery during a serious weather disturbance are in inverse proportion to the severity of his or her presenting illness or injury.

16. The chances of a blood-saturated sponge landing on your foot during surgery are inversely proportionate to the length of time you have owned the shoes you are wearing times the amount you paid for them.

Reprinted with permission from Journal of Nursing Jocularity, © 1994; 4(2):9.

THE ZEN OF PHARMACY

Jim Plagakis, RPh

"There's a woman on the phone who wants to be counseled about her dog." I looked up at the technician, sighed, and said, "Tell her I'm a pharmacist, not a veterinarian." I was busy trying to practice *The Zen of Pharmacy*, doing my absolute best to stay balanced during a very busy time, attempting to keep all of my juggling balls in the air. I didn't think I could handle one more thing, and it didn't need to be a counseling session about a dog.

"She says that she can't afford a vet." The tech gave me a look.

"Ask her what it's about."

"Something wrong with her dog's eye." The tech frowned at me. "She sounds like she's 100 years old, Jim. Have a heart."

"Put her on hold," I grumbled. If she was patient enough to wait while I finished what I was doing, I'd give her a minute. Her dog! What next? I've run my fingers through patients' hair looking for nits, had people lift up their shirts and ask me to look at various rashes. *I'm not a doctor. I do not diagnose.* Men have whispered questions to me about sexual difficulties in hopes of finding a miracle aphrodisiac. Gynecological questions seem to embarrass me more than the women asking them. I have advised teenage girls on birth control methods and even had an overweight woman ask me to look at the eruptions under her bra line. But the pharmacist as the *go-to guy* about a dog's health—this was a first.

Now, if you are going to be a serious practitioner of *The Zen of Pharmacy*, you have to allow for just about anything. The study of Zen in the art of pharmacy is really a miniature study of the art of patience and generosity. Working in a retail pharmacy—working well, caring—is to become part of a process, to achieve a sort of balance and an inner peace of mind right in the middle of a 300-prescription day, phones ringing, cranky customers, impatient doctors, and a down computer. It means getting the job done without that dry-mouth sense of falling behind and that heart-pumping urgency.

I will admit that I am consistently a failure at practicing *The Zen of Pharmacy*. That doesn't mean that I haven't had my winning days, hours stacked high when I have been able to detach myself from the epinephrine-pumping craziness and, like a kite in the wind, just go with the flow. I like those days. They are magical, and I invariably go home relaxed and energized. I didn't rush to keep up, and, amazingly, the work got done. I didn't take it too seriously and just let the tide rise around me. This is a healthy time in the drug-store. I call it *The Zen of Pharmacy*.

This day, I was so far out of balance that my teeter-totter had slammed to the ground. I picked up the telephone and heard a fragile, elderly voice at the other end. "My little Poochie's eye is filled with matter," she said. "Is there anything I can do?"

"I'm not a veterinarian," I said, a chill in my voice. I noticed that the technician had just accepted a stack of prescriptions from a patient. I was already a half-dozen behind.

"I know, dear," she said sweetly. "I can't afford a veterinarian, and I thought perhaps you could help me." She was asking for me to be nice to her.

I was. For some inexplicable reason, nothing mattered except this little old lady and Poochie. She had charmed me. I recommended that she get an OTC eyewash and see a veterinarian if that did not work. She brought me cookies a week later. The eyewash had worked. I suddenly realized that there is more to the practice of pharmacy than increasing its speed.

Reprinted with permission from Drug Topics, © 1998; 142(4):44.

STOP WORKING SO HARD. GET YOURSELF FIRED.

Campion Quinn, MD

Do you hate your job? Have your once-rosy views of medicine been quashed by demanding patients, bean-counting hospital administrators, and rampantly proliferating HMOs?

If you're like a growing number of physicians, you're yearning to commit professional hara-kiri, but you can't bring yourself to do it—or don't know how. Instead, you sit around waxing eloquent about your brother-in-law on Wall Street or your cousin the real estate broker.

"He makes a million a year and still gets to golf three times a week."

"She never had to go to medical school or stay awake all night patching up the survivors of a train wreck."

"I think his company even pays for his car. What does the hospital do for us?"

What's surprising is that, once we're finished complaining, we typically grab the next patient's chart and get back to work—sacrificing sleep, leisure time, and peace of mind to serve the very people who've drained the joy out of our lives.

Why do we physicians grumble so much, then do our work with such skill and diligence? After giving this matter a great deal of thought, I had an epiphany: Most of us, being gifted with intelligence and a peerless work ethic, have never failed miserably at anything that calls for smarts and perseverance. Unlike my college roommate, Sal, who flunked physical education (the first student to do so in our school's history) and refused to register for any course where the teacher gave homework, we doctors doggedly slogged our way through chemistry classes and advanced anatomy. At the same time, we did after-school research projects and hospital volunteer work, maintained 4.0 grade point averages, and studied for the MCATs.

Having survived all this—and residency, too—we're primed to keep scampering ahead, like a rabbit that has spotted a carrot in the distance. Indeed, the cathartic words "I quit" rarely cross a doctor's lips. And do you know any physicians who've been fired? Not many, I'll bet.

Not for you, the pleasures of being cut loose and suddenly finding yourself with endless hours of free time. Enough time to write the novel that's been kicking around in your head, to learn to play the guitar, to place your family crest atop Mount Everest. Yes, you can do these things, and more, but first you'll need to lose that job.

How? you ask. If you're self-employed, I can't help you; you simply must summon the courage to close up shop. But if you have an employer and can't bring yourself to quit, you have another option: Get fired. Here's a 10-step plan designed to free you from the rigors of full-time employment.

1. Spread rumors about the hospital's imminent closing and the CEO's unconscionable golden parachute.

2. During a fund-raising gala to honor your employer's biggest benefactor, stand on a chair and shout, "I hear his family made its money selling nuclear secrets to Third World countries."

3. Issue a memo to all nursing stations ordering high-colonic enemas on rhinoplasty patients. Sign the chief of surgery's name.

4. Crash your employer's computer system and alter the billing records. (You're not a skilled computer hacker? Hire one. You'll find them on any college campus.)

5. Deliver a lecture to the dictation pool entitled, "Carpal-tunnel syndrome: making someone pay." Give attendees the business cards of local ambulance chasers.

6. At opportune moments toss out comments like "I think washing your hands before seeing patients

Copyright [©] 1997 by Medical Economics. Reprinted by permission from Medical Economics Magazine; 74(12):199–201.

is a waste of time," "I might be a typhoid carrier," and "Dr. Jekyll is my hero."

7. Tell your boss that you'll be taking every second Tuesday off to meet with your parole officer.

8. Indulge in the garlic-rich and flatulence-producing foods you've been depriving yourself of. Now's the time for an up close conversation with your boss about your last performance appraisal.

9. Junk your conservative wardrobe. Find a local thrift shop that specializes in used clothing from the 1960s and '70s. Select a nice array of bell-bottoms, psychedelic shirts, and love beads. Mustard, rust, and robin's-egg blue are the colors of choice for the soon-to-be unemployed.

10. Get drunk and demand to operate on one of your patients immediately—even if he doesn't need surgery and you're not a surgeon.

Follow these steps diligently. I know it won't be easy. Years of self-discipline and rigorous training must be undone. I recommend "buddying" up with a reformed workaholic or, better yet, a professional loafer. (I believe Sal is available.) Your pal should be on call around the clock to help you through the first difficult months. So if, for example, you're seized by an irresistible urge to write an admission or read a medical journal, you can pick up the phone and call your buddy instead.

When you've reached the 10th step, reward yourself. Take some well-deserved vacation time, even if—especially if—you've used all yours already. And don't spoil the fun by revealing your plans to other staff members. Imagine the laughs when you don't show up for shifts or take call for several weeks.

There will be many distractions. You will, for instance, be tempted by hospital duties. Those are for other doctors. Treat orders to "conform" or "get with the program" with insouciance. Remember, you're trying to get fired, not rack up Brownie points.

When you deign to show up at work, you may hear rumors that your job is in jeopardy or termination is imminent. Don't rejoice just yet. Instead, brace yourself for the climactic moment when the director "calls you on the carpet" (a stained, threadbare spot that bears the marks of sweat, tears, and anxious, shuffling feet).

When you're escorted into the director's office, remember: Arrogance is in; contrition is out. Your body language should say, "Hey, jerk, you're interrupting my coffee break!" Act sullen and disrespectful, and don't let your guard down. These meetings have an ugly tendency to turn conciliatory. Generous offers may pour forth—paid leave, disability, even free psychiatric counseling.

To get the meeting back on track, let loose with one of the following bombshells: "Neglecting my patients? At least I'm not a necrophiliac like [state the director of pathology's name]"; or, "Me, lazy? Well, shouldn't [state the hospital or HMO president's name] be seeing that we physicians aren't overcharged for the cocaine that's sold in the laundry room?" Before the director can regain his composure, deliver the coup de grâce: Demand a huge salary increase. That ought to do it. You'll be fired.

Congratulations. Having gotten the boot, it's time to burn those bridges. Employment recidivism is epidemic among fired doctors, and you want to ensure that no one will offer you another job for quite some time.

First, no matter how generous your severance package, demand more. If they capitulate, ask for the furniture in the lobby and the right to house your visiting relatives in empty exam rooms. Insist that your former employers foot the bill for your retraining as a cheesemaker, rodeo clown, or vacuum-cleaner repairman. Once you're out the door, hold a press conference and reveal that patients are left to languish while pornographic movies—with colorful titles like "Doctor Octopus" and "Raunchy Rheumatologist"—are being shot in the doctors' lounge.

Your liberation is now complete. Tune up that guitar. Everest awaits. Oh, I suppose most of you will be employed again someday. But now you can console yourself in the knowledge that if you get another job you hate, losing it will be a breeze.

SPEAKING PATIENTLY

Taking great care of ourselves can only go so far, and eventually most folks will need to seek professional health care. What provider to choose and what regimen to follow is bewildering for patients as they are battered by conflicting information. It's not enough anymore for patients to be passive spectators, they are now expected to be largely responsible for their own health. No matter where on the health care food chain you live, patients are the premier reason for being in that profession. If ever there was time for sharing levity with patients, it's now.

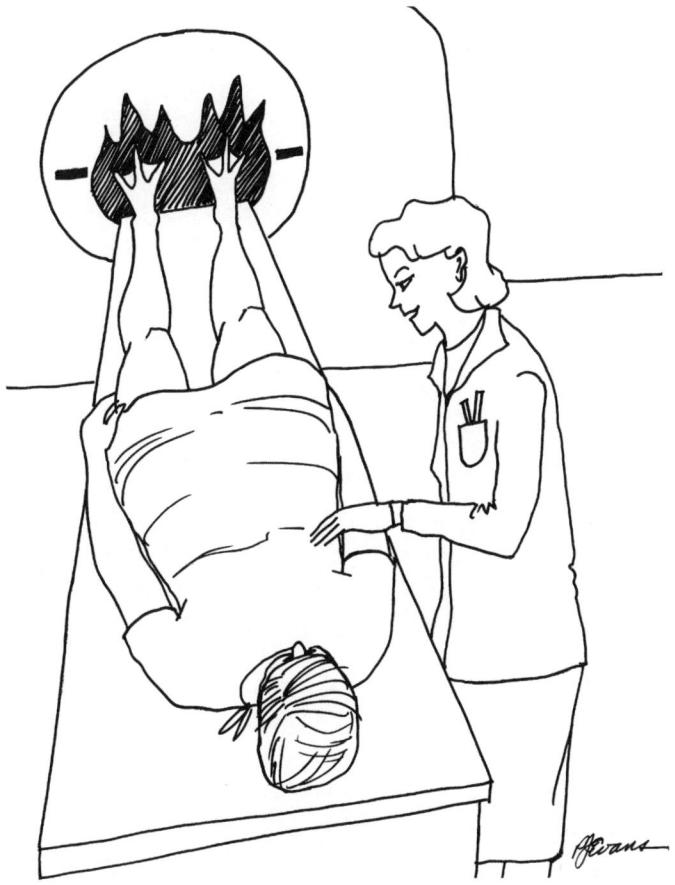

"Don't worry, Mr. Clancy, we've seen cases like yours before."

GONE FISHING

Jeannette Wolfe, MD

This past year a 3½-year-old child was brought into our department with a rather large fish hook embedded in his right thumb. He arrived by ambulance and when he was dropped off, the paramedics instructed me to ask the child what he caught fishing. The result is the following story.

Apparently, this was to be one of the child's first great bonding experiences with his dad as they were going bass fishing together for the first time. Dad left to get last-minute supplies (cold beer), briefly leaving the boy at home with mom and the fishing equipment. Well, the rods were rigged with lures large enough to snag Moby Dick. One end of the lure consisted of an orange plastic bobber the size of a small life preserver, and the other end had a labyrinthine barbed-hook system consisting of 3 large prongs each subdividing into 3 smaller prongs.

The immediate sequelae of the next series of events is somewhat vague. Mom, a nonfisherperson, was in another room happily preparing for her afternoon of child-free activity. Presumably, the family's black Lab, their pet parakeet, and the little boy were just *innocently* checking out the fishing equipment when the dog, Luke, mistook the lure for one of his squeeze toys and bit it. The hook snagged and actually went through the dog's mouth. Trying to help the dog, the little boy grabbed for the lure and got his thumb and palm caught in one of the other prongs. Now, dog and toddler are physically attached via the lure. There's more . . . next, the dog tried to swat the lure with his front leg, and the final prong got stuck in his paw. Mom runs in to find her son wailing, the dog yelping, and the parakeet maniacally flying above everyone. As the dog and the boy start a modified tug-of-war, mom tries to intervene. Unfortunately, it is quickly apparent to her that the hook and its company are not going to peacefully separate, and she looks around for help. Naturally, fisherman dad has yet to reappear, so she grabs the dog's chain—remember the dog is now hobbling on 3 legs—and her screaming child's shirt collar. The 3 of them hop, limp, and crawl to the phone in the next room (which mom swears is light years away) and mom dials 911.

EMS responded quickly and saved the day with a set of pliers. Dad arrived home just in time to take the dog and what was left of his decapitated lure to the vet. The dog eventually needed surgery to remove the hook from his mouth. Fortunately, the child fared better after a little bit of oral midazolam, a good digital block, and a Superman sticker.

In answer to my question as to what he caught fishing, the child's drugged eyes grew big. He enthusiastically spread his small arms out as wide as they could go and said in true fisherman style, "I caught Luke and he was this big!"

Reproduced from Annals of Emergency Medicine, © 1999; 33(4): 471–472, with permission from Mosby, Inc.

SIZZLING SECRET CLINICAL CONFESSIONS

Steven Tiger, PA

"Supervising Physician, forgive me, for I have sinned. Three times this past week. It's the usual thing. I'm still harboring *negative attitudes* about some of my patients. Not all of them, you understand, just some of them.

"I don't mean nice patients like Ms. A. She presented with a terse and precise history, cooperated with the physical examination, laboratory studies and other investigations, asked a few intelligent questions, and then cleared out of my office on schedule. The diagnosis was an acute, easily correctable condition. She complied with treatment and the outcome was excellent. All in all, a perfect clinical experience. Honestly, I wish some of my problem cases were more like Ms. A.

"I mean problem cases like Mr. Z. 'The Patient From Hell,' we call him. The bane of our practice. His complaints are always vague, rambling and unreliable. He's demanding and resentful, clingy and noncompliant. There has never been any clear diagnosis, but he keeps coming back . . . and back . . . and back. . . . Each session with him takes twice as long as the time scheduled, and he keeps phoning me at the worst times to ask the most asinine questions. When I was a student, one of my preceptors assigned a really irritating patient to me. And sometimes I think, 'Wouldn't it be nice to have an eager student around right now, to take Mr. Z off my hands, at least for awhile?'

"Last week, when I confessed this same sin, Supervising Physician, you told me to perform three fecal disimpactions as an act of contrition. I did, and I felt better for awhile. But I still keep wishing I didn't have to deal with Mr. Z."

Pride and Prejudice

Being a professional doesn't mean having no attitudes. It means not letting attitudes interfere with clinical responsibilities. Unfortunately, sometimes attitudes do interfere. Certain types of patients are just not high on the list of clinicians' favorites: patients with chronic progressive or terminal illness, the moribund elderly, and drug addicts to name some obvious examples.

It's confession time, so let's be honest. More often than not, students and graduates alike would rather see pleasant and otherwise-healthy patients with readily curable problems than the institutionalized elderly, the chronically ill, the psychiatrically disturbed or the developmentally disabled. And poor Mr. Z will never win any popularity awards.

Are you offended by this idea? Why? It is not a criticism of those patients. Their needs are real and they deserve the same quality of care as any other patients receive. Nor is it a slight against clinicians who choose to work with those patients. On the contrary, it is a sobering observation of a widely held attitude within the clinical professions. Take a poll of your classmates or colleagues and ask how many of them would *like* to work in a nursing home, for example, even at a slight increase in salary. Not many—*q.e.d.*

A professional takes pride in doing a job successfully. The problem with "problem patients" is that the usual criteria of success are seldom achieved, and the clinician's pride suffers when confronted by what looks like failure. It is a prejudice stemming from our orientation toward acute treatment and cure. The result of this prejudice is avoidance of those very patients whose problems have no quick and easy cure.

A Subtler Form of Avoidance

The Patient From Hell may be an exceptional case; a more common example of what many clinicians would rather avoid is the patient with emotional

Reprinted from Physician Assistant, © 1991; 15(6):8,13, with permission of the author.

problems. In school, relatively little attention is paid to such problems as anxiety and depression, beyond the self-evident observation that serious illness is a stressful experience and some platitudes about being understanding and sensitive toward patients. The curriculum rarely covers these subjects in anywhere near the depth that "real" medical topics like cardiology are covered. Consequently, many practitioners still do not realize that problems like anxiety and depression often have a physiologic origin; that the diagnostic criteria for these problems are clear and specific; and that there are effective treatments beyond counseling. In this case, it is the lack of familiarity that breeds contempt.

Be honest. Did you find the lectures on psychiatric problems as alluring and exciting as the material on emergency medicine and surgery? *Honestly?* These attitudes stem from the very orientation of clinical education, which seems to be based on a definition of success as portrayed on television shows in which the heroic doctor saves the patient in 30 or 60 minutes minus time for commercials.

The bad news is that some clinicians have an attitude problem. The good news is that most of those same clinicians try not to let their attitudes affect their clinical practice. The best news would be that such attitudes are disappearing—which should be one of the goals of education.

PRE-OP INSTRUCTIONS AS OUR PATIENTS HEAR THEM

March Warn, RN

Diet and NPO Instructions

Surgery can be a stressful experience. It is necessary that you prepare your body for this experience by providing the necessary fuel. We suggest that on the way into the hospital you stop and have a hearty breakfast. Steak and eggs, hash browns, biscuits and gravy, at least two cups of coffee and a large orange juice should see you through your surgical experience.

If your child is scheduled for surgery, he or she will likely be cranky on the trip into the hospital. Stop at a convenience store and get a large Coke and a Twinkie to settle your child down.

Clothing/Makeup

Since you will be seen by a large number of people while in our waiting room, we suggest that you dress up in your finest clothing and jewelry. Do not forget to apply a full coat of makeup, since you probably look sickly without it. If you are scheduled for a gynecological procedure be sure to wear pantyhose and a girdle. Several thicknesses of a bright nail polish will impress the surgical team with your fashion sense. And, so the admitting nurse will have no questions about your ability to pay your bill, wear every piece of jewelry you own.

Children scheduled for surgery should be dressed in the finest clothing, preferably bought just for this occasion, especially if they are going to have a tonsillectomy or tooth extraction. Large, heavy shoes with hard, sharp soles will help keep their feet warm in the recovery room. Be sure to tie the laces in complex knots so your child cannot remove them easily.

Arrival Time

We will give you a time when you should arrive at the hospital. However, since hospitals, like doctors'

Reprinted with permission from Journal of Nursing Jocularity, © 1996; 6(4):22–23. Edited from the original.

offices, always run late, it is best to arrive at least two hours after that appointment time. This will prevent a long, boring session in our waiting room.

Diagnostic Test Results

If your referring doctor has given you copies of any diagnostic tests he or she may have performed at their office, do not bring these with you. We have a fax machine and our secretary really enjoys calling doctors' offices to have test results faxed over. (We don't think she ever gets any good mail at home, so this is very exciting for her.)

Home Medications

If you are taking any medications at home on a regular basis we would like to know about them. It is not necessary for you to know the name or your dose of these medications. Just a general description will do. For instance, you can tell us that you take half a pink football, two plain round white pills and a speckled capsule at breakfast and the rest of the pink football at bedtime. We will know exactly what you are taking since we are trained professionals and can identify all medications by their color and shape.

Past Medical/Surgical History

It is not necessary for you to know detailed information about your medical history. Just tell us you have had "stomach trouble" or that sometime in the past, a doctor once said you had "a funny heart sound."

And, if you have ever had relatives whose surgery was canceled because they ran very high fevers after they were given anesthesia, don't tell us or we might cancel your surgery and you will have taken a day off from work for nothing.

We don't need to know that you bleed for several hours any time you cut yourself shaving, or that you bruise easily. All surgical patients are going to bleed anyway.

You need not tell us about your surgical history. If you can't remember whether you have had your gallbladder, appendix, uterus or ovaries removed, don't worry. One of our favorite OR games is called "guess the surgery." After you are asleep, we try to guess which organs you have had removed by interpreting the scars on your body. And if you can't remember which side your hernia, breast lump, lipoma, or varicose vein is on, we will simply make an educated guess. We have a 50-50 chance of being correct.

Transportation

You will likely be given lots of narcotic and anesthetic agents while you are in surgery. After surgery, you may be drowsy or have diminished reflexes. You wouldn't want any of your family members or friends to see you in this condition, so drive yourself to the hospital and do not make arrangements for anyone to drive you home. After all, once you get out of the city, it is a straight shot up the interstate to your house.

MY DOG ATE MY RUNNING SHOES

Fitness Excuses From Patients

Amber Stenger

Excuses, excuses. You've probably heard hundreds of them from patients about why they don't exercise. Here's a sample of some of our favorites from friends of THE PHYSICIAN AND SPORTSMEDICINE.

Think you've heard it all? Has one of your patients ever invoked fears of grizzly bears or "hyenas" as reasons for not exercising? How about volcanic ash or earthquakes?

As your patients file into your office this month, many will come armed with a New Year's resolve to lose weight, start exercising, and eat right. But by next month, their conviction may have dissolved, replaced by excuses for not upholding their health resolutions.

To help you keep your sense of humor, we asked several physicians about some of the more outrageous fitness excuses they've heard from patients. If your patients use any excuse from the list below, you will be able to tell them that you *have* heard it before.

"I can't exercise because I'm out of shape."

"I can't exercise because of the grizzly bear," which was sighted near a popular walking path.

"Well, if I go and exercise, any time that I will live longer I will have spent exercising, and therefore I will have wasted it."

"My hair might get messed up."

"Exercise makes the hair on my legs grow, and it hurts."

"I would have exercised, but there was a war."

"An earthquake drained my pool."

"I only have so many heart beats left, and I don't want to waste them on exercise."

"My mother told me not to jog because my uterus would fall out."

"I can't. I have a hyena."

"My previous doctor told me it wasn't good for me."

"I don't want to break a nail."

"My wife would be angry with me if I lost weight."

"Why would I exercise if I don't have to?"

"Working out makes my boyfriend jealous."

"I can't because of the volcanic ash."

"I don't want to give my mother the satisfaction of saying I'm taking care of myself."

"If I exercise, I might not have enough energy left over for sex."

"I hate to sweat."

"My rollerblades are broken."

"My kids would laugh at me."

"I forgot my workout clothes."

"The TV at the gym is always on something I don't want to watch."

"I'm afraid I won't remember my locker number."

"My thong [leotard] shrank."

"All they sell to eat is health food."

Some of the best reasons patients have missed their physical therapy appointments through the years at the Orthopaedic Center of the Rockies in Fort Collins, Colorado:

"Had cow poo all over."

"Had to go to Disneyland."

"Had Final Four tickets."

"Cops stopped by to haul me in for check fraud."

Reprinted with permission of McGraw-Hill, Inc. from The Physician and Sportsmedicine, © 1993; 21(1):149–150.

NOT JUST WINDOW DRESSING:

Gowns as the Latest Fashion
Pam Johnson, BS, RT(R)

The door opens and onto the fashion runway steps—a patient. What that patient wears leaving the dressing room may surprise you. The classic medical joke from cartoons to get-well cards features the patient gown.

We offer two gowns to patients undergoing x-rays, other than chest and extremity, along with the instructions, "Please put these on in opposite directions," or "Put these on with one open in back and one in front." A patient's interpretation of those instructions often results in a fashion show.

The most prevalent runway activity involves two no-change changes—the patient who appears wearing a gown or two over clothes and the person who opens the changing room door with nothing on.

Others wear only one gown, open in back or front. We hear, "I thought you made a mistake," "I don't need two gowns," or "I thought you meant to give me pants."

Women appreciate a reminder to use the second gown.

Men present another challenge. If they can be convinced to use the dressing room at all, they usually resist the two-gown idea, preferring the open back. Some men don't fathom that other patients can't appreciate the view, even as the audience turns away in embarrassment.

Next down the runway come variations on the theme "tied at the back." The gown is tied at the neck like a bib, leaving the sleeves empty. Scanning down, the gown's neck can be seen, tied under the arms or at the waist. The gown may be open in front or at the side, sarong-like.

One man wore the second gown tied in the front with the hem pulled between his legs and the material tucked in at the waist, creating shorts.

I've witnessed heads poking through armholes in an asymmetric fashion that would make designer Issai Miyake proud.

One woman donned a gown, front open, and sat in the waiting room using the other gown as a blanket—over her legs.

Some patients put both gowns on the same way so that they gape revealingly open. These patients often claim that they thought we gave them just another dumb hospital instruction.

We always are alert for the patients, usually men, who disrobe with the door open, if they are not allowed to undress in the hall. When women do this, they laugh in embarrassment at the way the hospital makes them lose all modesty.

Men give me mock looks of disappointment, like I'm ruining their fun.

People frequently enter the exam room and start to shed their gowns. They look amazed when we ask them not to disrobe and often comment, "X-rays can go through this?"

I can't believe that they seem to believe their bodies are less dense than thin cloth.

Our department once used three-armhole wrap-around gowns that seemed less confusing and provided more coverage than our present styles. Like a tasty item at a local restaurant, good things usually are discontinued.

I'm waiting for the day a patient puts his legs through armholes like pants.

Fortunately, at the end of a day we can't bow and take credit for our patients' creativity, like fashion designers do at the end of a show. But some Paris designers might wish they could.

Reprinted from ASRT Scanner, © 1998; 30(10):32, with permission of the author.

UNRECALLED FALLS

Jeff Brone

On November 1, 1995, the *Arkansas Journal of Medicine* reported that one out of every five people does not remember having fallen down a flight of stairs. This article is on the heels of the reports from Darris Solvang, a noted hypnotherapist and meat inspector of Skyridge, WY, who has helped many of his patients recall long repressed episodes of falling down stairs. A disturbing trend, or a long overdue problem.

It's true. You may have fallen down a whole flight of stairs and not even remember it. Call it Selective Trauma Affective Internalized Repression Syndrome, or STAIRS for short, and it can affect anyone. Daniel Truesdale, an acute sufferer, was once rolled down 150 foam rubber stairs (for his own safety), and only could recall three of them (numbers 5, 74 and 108). There are several reasons why you might not remember such an encounter:

1. You're really, really preoccupied.

2. You're a senior citizen. Your memory might be failing, and selectively your brain remembers only vital information, like who didn't call you on your birthday, while forgetting things like falling and the like.

3. You have associated it with a childhood trauma and blocked it out. This one is usually most lucrative for the hypnotherapist.

Dr. Robert Narry, of the National Falling Down Institute in Darbyville, GA, makes the point that people should not be overly alarmed by this syndrome. There is every chance that you haven't fallen down stairs recently. He offered this simple advice in his latest symposium entitled "The Humpty Dumpty Syndrome." He urged us to ask ourselves these questions. A yes answer may mean that something is wrong:

Are people saying things like "Are you OK?" and "Nice tumble there, Wallenda" and "You clumsy imbecile"?

Do you have unexplained bruises, head pains and the urge to be "helped up"?

When you get to the bottom of some stairs, do you break into an uncontrollably joyful version of Barry Manilow's "Looks Like We Made It"?

When descending stairs, do people insist that you "go first"?

If you answered yes to any of these questions, you may have fallen down stairs recently. If so, there is a chance to bring back the memory and make peace with the stairs down which you fell. The institute has established a hotline; 1-800-555-I Think I Broke Something. Operators can suggest doctors and things. Call. There's nothing to be afraid of—except stairs. You clod.

Reprinted with permission from Journal of Irreproducible Results, © 1996; 41(1):4.

FINDING HUMOR IN OUR WORKPLACE

Sharon P. Hall, RNC

In my 30 years as a perinatal nurse, I've collected or heard some terrifically funny tales about us, our patients, and the services that we perform. And sharing them with others is especially fun. Here goes:

Par for the Course

A childbirth educator relays the story of a room full of pregnant women and their partners for a Lamaze class. The instructor was teaching the women how to breathe properly, along with informing all of the partners how to give the necessary assurances at this stage of the plan.

The educator then announced, "ladies, exercise is good for you. Walking is especially beneficial. And gentlemen, it wouldn't hurt you to take the time to go walking with your partner!" The room got really quiet. Finally, a man in the middle of the group raised his hand and asked, "Is it all right if she carries a golf bag while we walk?" Yeah, right!

The Right Word, Please

As perinatal nurses, we are often amused when patients tell us they would like "their epidermal" (epidural) or that they "are here this morning to be seduced!" (induced). I will always remember the look on one mother's face when my colleague told her "the baby will be placed under the hood."

It's also been related to me that there were two 10-year-old boys who were overheard discussing birth at the entrance to the LDRP suite, and one said, "They call it a delivery room, but it's really a take-out place." One pediatric nurse overheard a little girl tell her brother in the waiting room, "He gave me a shot for the mumps, measles, and rebellion." And last, there was that time when I went to give a fetal monitoring lecture at a local hotel and the marquee read "fatal monitoring."

Charting Chuckles

The strangest things get written down in our effort to tell the whole story of the women for whom we provide care. Describing a woman recovering from an epidural, one nurse wrote, "the left leg remains numb at times, but she walked it off." Or "at the time of pregnancy, the woman was undergoing bronchoscopy." I once read, "she was treated with Mycostatin or suppositories." Or how about, "both the patient and myself report the passing of flatus."

One nurse wrote, "the patient has contractions if she lies on her right side for several months." One admission was noted as "healthy-appearing, decrepit 69-year-old female, mentally alert but forgetful." And finally, "The pelvic examination was done on the floor." I once wrote, "the patient was admitted to the hospital on the day of admission." I left it just to see if anyone would notice—and of course, no one did!

I've also seen some good stuff written by our medical colleagues: "We have been sitting on this patient for some time." How about, "this unfortunate 60-year-old woman has been seen by me for 10 years." Also, "patient was dismissed home without dressing"; "Mrs. Jones was admitted with diarrhea from the ER"; and "the patient has never been pregnant and denies any reason for this."

Women Say the Funniest Things

One nurse related that she gave a woman a referral slip for the GI clinic. The woman stated,

"This must be wrong, I was never in the military service." A nurse fielding a phone call from an anxious lady was asked, "How long does it take to get over gamma globulin?"

Reprinted with permission from AWHONN Lifelines, © 1998; 2(6):64,63.

One woman, waking up from general anesthesia in the recovery room, was told by the nurse, "You have a beautiful baby boy!" The mother said, "I do? Well, what is his name?" This one from a frail, elderly lady on admission: "I've been in this hospital so often, it's like home. I know everyone. What's your name?"

Overheard in the surgical suite: "Why can't I wear lipstick to surgery? I'm having my uterus removed, not my lips!" One primiparous woman after unloading two suitcases, a video camera, two still cameras, a "goody bag," and a potpourri pot, smiled and joyfully stated, "My contractions are 15 minutes apart, I think I'm in labor."

An elderly lady, being questioned by a nurse regarding her activity, reported, "lately, I've gotten into transcendental vegetation."

A patient once told me that she had been having repeated bouts of Braxton-Hicks contractions in her 39th week of pregnancy. One night, as she tossed and turned in discomfort, her husband turned over and, placing his mouth very close to her abdomen, stated, "Stay in your womb and don't come out until we tell you."

You Know It's Been A Bad Day When . . .

- The nurse manager says, "we have a few changes . . ."
- No one shows for mother-baby class
- Your patient passes out in the bathroom after a Fleets enema, and you gently slide her down your legs where she sits on your shoes
- You drop your pager in the toilet

MANDATORY INFECTION OUT-OF-CONTROL TEST

Steven J. Schweon
Eileen O'Rourke
Susan Trout
Robert Quinn-O'Connor
Elaine Neely

The Joint Commission on Accreditation of Healthcare Organizations mandates yearly infection control in-service programs for all clinical personnel. At times, these live presentations or written tests can be tedious and repetitive. We may lose our targeted audience to the land of zzzzz's. As an exciting alternative, we offer a written test that will stimulate the cerebral cortex and still fulfill the Joint Commission requirements. The questions and answers have been proven to be statistically significant, by mischievous, complex, and perplexing analytical tools (to be publicized at an upcoming media gala). One word of caution, pneumocraniums (air-heads) need not bother to take this grueling examination. Choose the best answer:

1. Frank Pus is:
   a. A reclusive wild man in Montana
   b. The man who developed the hit "Puss 'N Boots"
   c. An alternative rock group

2. Your patient has been diagnosed with Ebola. You:
   a. Run like crazy
   b. Delegate care to others so they may acquire first-hand experience
   c. Ponder your life expectancy

Reproduced from American Journal of Infection Control, © 1998; 26(4):449–450, with permission from Mosby Year Book, Inc.

3. Kuru is:
   a. The next dance craze
   b. A tropical fruit
   c. A political uprising

4. Mad cow disease has resulted in:
   a. Bovine Prozac
   b. Cows with self-esteem issues
   c. Udderly disgraceful British scientists milking the hysteria

5. Infectious humor
   a. Should be isolated
   b. Can be contagious
   c. Is reportable to local health departments

6. Vampires should:
   a. Be aware of their victim's HIV, HBV status
   b. Substitute tomato juice for blood when thirsty
   c. Consult a psychiatrist

7. Urotherapy is drinking your urine for health (true!). Public health implications include:
   a. Replacement of Listerine in fighting germs
   b. 12-step group formation for those who are addicted
   c. Replacing beer as the beverage of choice for many Americans
   d. Food and Drug Administration regulation

8. Before administering a lethal injection to a prisoner, you must:
   a. Clean the skin with alcohol
   b. Use a sterile syringe
   c. Prepare and administer using strict aseptic technique
   d. All of the above

9. Bacteria
   a. Is the back exit of a cafeteria
   b. Are sexually active, hedonistic little guys
   c. Keep us employed

10. Microbiologists enjoy:
    a. Multiple organisms
    b. Watching asexual reproduction
    c. Being peeping toms in the micro world

11. Sex is the leading cause of STD.
    a. True
    b. False

12. Sal Monella is:
    a. A street vendor
    b. A man who resides in Italy
    c. A fish that swims upstream

13. Universal precautions is:
    a. Practiced at Universal Studios, Hollywood
    b. Being cautious when working out on a Universal weight-lifting machine
    c. Also practiced by the shuttle astronauts

14. Cherpies is a STD transmitted by birds, but is tweatable.
    a. True
    b. False

15. If Goldilocks had chickenpox, would you isolate the 3 bears?
    a. Yes
    b. No

16. Does the old woman who lives in a shoe with her 13 children need antifungal foot powder?
    a. Yes
    b. No

17. Roofers are prone to shingles.
    a. True
    b. False

18. The foremost in airborne precautions include:
    a. Holding your breath
    b. Wearing a NASA prototype space suit
    c. Leaving the health care profession

19. Aerobic bacteria have low resting heart rates and are generally healthy.
    a. True
    b. False

20. "Looking for pus in all the wrong places" best describes the work of infection control.
    a. True
    b. False

21. Maltophilia is:
    a. An affinity for malted milkshakes
    b. Prince's real name
    c. An island off the coast of Italy

22. Does the playing and dancing to the "Chicken Song" at weddings foster chickenpox transmission?
    a. Yes
    b. No

23. *Providencia stuartii* is the yearly meeting of the Stuartii family in Rhode Island.
    a. True
    b. False

24. Using a finger cot while picking your nose will prevent bacterial self-inoculation.
    a. True
    b. False

25. Cellular reproduction:
    a. Takes place in jails only
    b. Describes the increase in cellular phones
    c. Is the cloning of sales people

26. Staph is found
    a. On sheet music
    b. With serpents
    c. Never in a store when you need help

27. Hepatitis is known to be highly communicable at HEP rallies.
    a. True
    b. False

28. Surgical scrubbing, which kills zillions of bacteria on an international level, is synonymous with mass murdering.
    a. True
    b. False

29. The cure for hepatitis does NOT involve a mostly liquid diet followed by singing many choruses of "HEP, HEP, Hooray."
    a. True
    b. False

30. Describe the best disinfection method if the guillotine was brought back for capital punishment:
    a. Just change the blade daily
    b. Why bother?

31. *Aspergillus* is the snake that bit Cleopatra.
    a. True
    b. False

32. A spirochete is a tropical bird that flies in circles.
    a. True
    b. False

33. The favorite movie of Centers for Disease Control and Prevention epidemiologists is:
    a. Germs of Endearment
    b. One Flu Over the Cuckoo's Nest
    c. The Germinator
    d. "Bugs" Bunny and Elmer Blood

JUST A NUMBER, OR IS IT?

Cliff Thomas, RPh

I hired a young first-year pharmacy student for the summer months to give him some practical exposure to the profession. On his first day, I lectured him about being friendly and professional. I instructed him to be available to the customer and to open the door of communication with the customer whenever possible.

We had a very good customer from the retirement complex who was proud of her youthful appearance. She tried very hard to project the image of being younger than her years.

On a July morning during a sequence of record-breaking high temperatures, our retired customer entered our pharmacy and headed for the prescription counter. As she approached my new "eager to please" potential pharmacist, she wiped her brow, smiled, and said, "Going to be 102 today." He returned her smile and said, "Happy Birthday!"

Reprinted with permission from Drug Topics, © 1998; 142(2):47.

THE DRAG AND NAG METHOD OF GAIT TRAINING

Martha Somers, PT

We've all seen it. At some point, many of us have done it. The Drag and Nag (D & N) method of gait training is alive and well. Yet in physical therapy literature, education, and continuing education, scant attention is paid to this unique approach to the restoration of ambulatory abilities. Since D & N is such a prevalent practice, it deserves a closer look.

Drag and Nag may be one of the oldest restorative techniques, dating back to pre-historic times. Paintings depicting D & N have been discovered on the walls of caves in southwestern France. (These figures have also been interpreted to be representations of fertility rites.) During the crusades, Teutonic knights are known to have practiced D & N as they assisted fallen comrades from fields of battle.

In modern times, the Drag and Nag method of gait training has alternately been referred to as "maximal assist ambulation" and "passive ambulation." In its most basic form, D & N consists of dragging a patient up and down the parallel bars while nagging him about his gait pattern. A variation of the technique involves dragging the patient back and forth outside of the parallel bars, pushing along a walker in front. Drag and Nag is most effective when carried out by multiple therapists, each pulling on a different body part.

Typical commands given during Drag and Nag therapy include "Take a step," "Take some of your weight," or the ultimate of D & N commands, "Put your feet on the floor." A well-coordinated team of therapists will issue multiple commands at once, with each therapist talking about a different action. This approach is most effective if the commands conflict.

Whether the uni- or multi-therapist approach is used, many therapists find it useful to augment the treatment with threats. The therapist may threaten not to allow the patient to return to his room, or vow to send him to a nursing home if he doesn't cooperate. A more imaginative therapist may threaten to steal the hospital gown.

The advantages of Drag and Nag therapy are obvious. Unfortunately, the Drag and Nag approach to gait training has one minor flaw: it is of no benefit to the patient.

Reprinted from *The Neurology Report*, © 1993; 17(1):26, with permission of the Neurology Section, APTA. Edited from the original.

BUGS ARE NOT FUNNY SYNDROME

Steven J. Schweon, RN, MPH
Ellen Novatnack, RN, BSN
Eileen O'Rourke, MT (ASCP), CIC
Susan Trout, RN, CIC

To the Editor:

The recent identification of vancomycin-intermediate *Staphylococcus aureus* has reinvigorated legitimate fears in the infection control community that the microbe world is going amuck. This has had a dramatic impact on the behavior of a few of our fellow infection control professionals. Signs and symptoms include the following:

1. Contemplating a telephone condom for your office;
2. Taking a shower with a mask on to prevent legionnaire's disease;
3. Installing sinks at the front door so guests can wash before entering;
4. Washing your hands before and after going to the bathroom, just in case;
5. Demanding that waiters wash their hands before serving meals (and observing them do so);
6. Keeping a bottle of disinfectant spray handy to use on hand-held items between use;
7. Removing all blenders from your home;
8. Always carrying an extra pen in case someone asks to borrow one, so you can say, "keep it, I have an extra";
9. Requiring sedation when someone in an elevator sneezes without covering his or her mouth;
10. Always being prepared by carrying a "sinkless" handwashing agent wherever you go;
11. Placing handwashing stickers in your home bathroom as a reminder for family members and guests to wash up;
12. Waking up in a cold sweat from a nightmare involving mouth pipetting, eating, and drinking in the laboratory;
13. Development of rage attacks when making rounds and seeing a patient in Contact Precautions for methicillin-resistant coagulase-negative staphylococci.

Reprinted with permission from Infection Control and Hospital Epidemiology, © 1999; 20(8):527.

TRADING PLACES

The myth of immunity states that health providers are simply not allowed to ever get sick themselves. It's fairly easy to ignore early signs of illness and continue to be care givers rather than care receivers. At some point though, denial will no longer work and the professional reluctantly learns to switch roles. Procedures that were always described to patients as being minor, suddenly don't seem so minor when they are happening to you. For a crash course in empathy, there's nothing quite like the experience of being a patient. By the way, when was your last check-up?

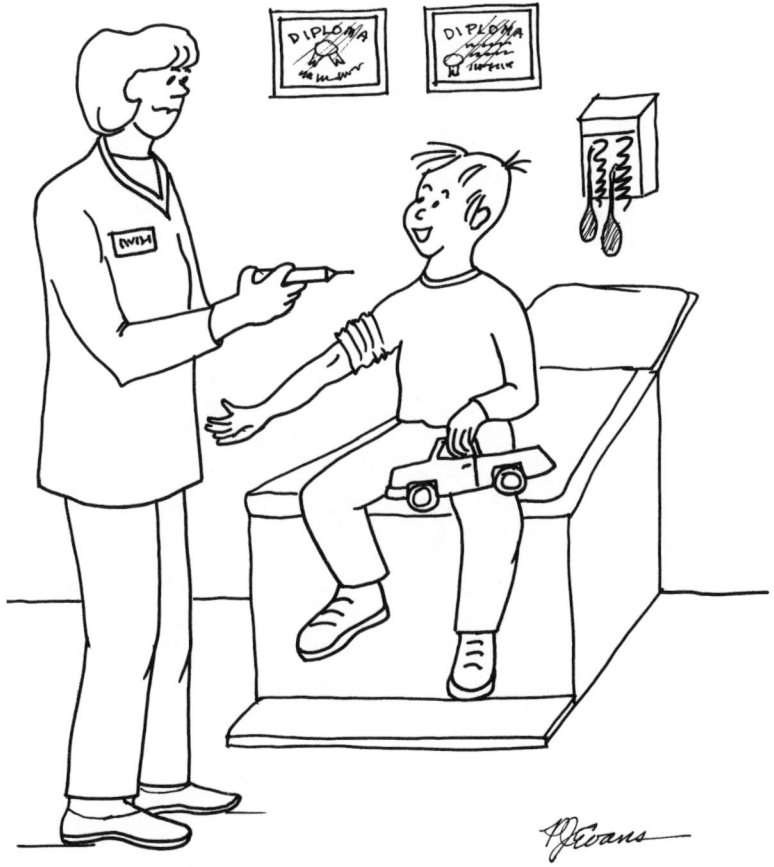

"How about I give you the shot and you play with the truck?"

HOW TO VISIT THE DOCTOR

Howard J. Bennett, MD

Countless numbers of children are wheeled, walked, or driven to doctors' offices every day. Here's some advice on how to visit the doctor—from the child's point of view.

Going to the Office

Hide in your bedroom when your mother tells you it's time to leave for your checkup. Ignore her when she calls you for the second time. As soon as you hear her coming up the stairs, shout that you don't feel well and would rather stay home. Get dressed in a hurry when you see that she's really mad.

Stop to tie your shoelace on the way to the car. While you're kneeling down, admire the grass stains on your brand-new sneakers. Then stand up and look upset. When your mother says, "What's wrong now?" state that you left Fred (your teddy bear) inside. Plan on taking ten minutes to find him. Do it in five when your mother tells you it's now or else.

As the car pulls away, tell your mother you love her a lot. Tell her she's the best mom in the whole world. In the whole galaxy. In the whole universe. Ask if you can stop at McDonald's. When she says no, explain that it's not for you, but for Fred. Do not be reassured when she says Fred can wait until after your checkup.

In the Waiting Room

Walk two steps behind your mother as you approach the check-in area. Ask her if you can play with the toys. As you walk over to the play area, stare at the other children. Ask one of the boys why he came to the doctor's office. Announce that you are perfect and only need a checkup. Agree to have a contest to see who is the strongest. Compare muscles. Compare stomachs. Compare who can jump the highest. Compare who can hold his breath the longest. Look a little worried when his mother comes to take him in to see the doctor. Declare yourself the champion.

Find the play doctor's kit. Open it and check to see if any of the pieces are missing. Put the stethoscope around your neck. Take your temperature. Take Fred's temperature. Find the biggest needle and tell Fred he has to get a shot. Say, "It won't hurt," and then jab it into his arm. Repeat five times, then look around to see if anyone was watching. Smile at your mom. Give Fred a kiss.

In the Exam Room

After the nurse records your height and weight, ask if it's time to go home. When your mother comments that the doctor hasn't seen you yet, ignore her. Look around the room. Leave Fred on the paper-lined examination table as you hop down to check things out. Look at each of the instruments hanging on the wall. Ask what the blood-pressure cuff is for. Ask what the ophthalmoscope is for. Ask what the rubber hammer is for.

Open up one of the drawers under the examination table and pull out a plastic speculum. Decide it's a toy gun and shoot Fred. Point it at your mom and say, "Stick 'em up!" Act surprised when she hollers, "Where did you get that from?" Frown when she tells you to stop playing with the doctor's equipment, sit down, and behave yourself.

Sit down next to your mother. Fold your hands in your lap and look guilty. After a minute or so, ask if you can get up and look around some more. Promise you'll be careful. Put on the cute smile you know she can't resist. As you wander around the room, pretend you don't hear when your mother reminds you not to touch anything.

Stand in front of the counter where the doctor keeps his medical supplies. Notice the funny smell. Try to avoid the odor by breathing through your mouth instead of your nose. Grip the counter and stand on your tiptoes so you can see all the way to

Reproduced with permission from *The Journal of Family Practice*, © 1997; 44(5):507–508.

the back. Count the Band-Aids. Count the Q-Tips. Wonder if cotton balls and cotton candy are the same thing. Find the jar where the tongue depressors are kept. As you take one from the middle, lose your balance so the rest end up on the floor. When the doctor enters the room, stop whatever you are doing, grab Fred, and hide under your mother's chair. She will probably say something like, "Oh, so now you need me."

Pretend you're not listening when the doctor compliments you on your sneakers. Suddenly become interested when he asks how Fred is. Smile when he feels a hot dog in Fred's stomach and sees birds in Fred's ears. Relax. Come out from under the chair and let the doctor examine you. Fiddle with your belly button as he listens to your heart. Giggle when he checks your reflexes. Be unable to stick out your tongue, no matter how many times he shows you how to say "Ah!"

After the doctor finishes examining you, ask if you are going to get a shot. If he says yes, announce that you have to go to the bathroom. Repeat five times, even though your mother will say that you'll have to wait. Kick and scream just before the needle goes in, but get your composure back as soon as you are given a Band-Aid. When the doctor offers you a lollipop, ask if Fred can have one too.

As you leave the office, allow your mother to convince you to say thank you to the doctor. Be glad that you got out alive. Remind your mom that she said you could go to McDonald's.

THE 12 PUFFS OF CHRISTMAS

Warren McNab

On the first day of Christmas, my cigarettes gave to me
A whole lot of agony
2nd day—Lots of stinky clothes
3rd day—Yellow teeth and fingers
4th day—Two lungs with cancer
5th day—Leu Ko Pla Kia
6th day—Ashtray-tasting kisses
7th day—Stressful nonstop air flights
8th day—Chronic emphysema
9th day—Coughing family members
10th day—Richer thoracic surgeons
11th day—Terminal carcinoma
12th day—Mourners singing softly

This article is reprinted with permission from the Journal of Health Education, Nov/Dec 1992:435. The Journal of Health Education is a publication of the American Alliance for Health, Physical Education, Recreation and Dance, 1900 Association Drive, Reston, Virginia 22091.

LEARNING TO WAIT WITH DIGNITY

Valentine Cardinale

If anyone needs to learn how to wait, it's yours truly. Patience is not one of my strongest traits. I've tended to avoid lines of all shapes, whatever they're for—tickets for the hottest movie of the year, the biggest buffet in the country, or the greatest giveaway since Chick-Fil-A.

I've gotten better over the years, however. Maybe that's because of all the sacrifice I went through during the 1980s, when I purposely waited on lines in department stores and supermarkets in a fit of self-improvement. Perhaps I'm just mellowing.

Today, I can wait on a runway if my plane is missing a part the pilot says it needs. I don't have to trim the bushes around my home in one day anymore; I do the front one week, the back a week or two later. I really don't mind waiting for my local news anchor to stop talking about Bill and Monica, so I can get the Yankees score and see whether Mark or Ken or Sammy hit one out.

Living in New Jersey—one of the most densely peopled states in the country—helps. The traffic is hot and heavy everywhere, even in the driveway, which now shelters cars for everyone in the family, so Jerseyites are almost used to someone breathing down their necks.

Which brings me to health care.

The wait time in the doctor's office is notoriously lengthy, but few people, if any, complain about it. They sit, silent sufferers, and wait and wait and wait. Recently, a woman in a doctor's waiting room I shared had had enough and started erupting:

"This is ridiculous. Two hours, I've been waiting. What does the doctor do: Take a break after seeing each patient?"

"It won't be long now," replied one of the assistants behind the front desk.

"It's like this every time now," continued Ms. Vesuvius. "I'll give it five more minutes. When I see the doctor, I'm going to tell him I'm going to start smoking again as soon as I leave the office."

"And who will you be hurting by doing that?" said another woman patient softly.

Emboldened by that remark, I added, "He's really a very good doctor. He takes the time to talk with each patient, and you don't see enough of that these days." The soft-spoken woman nodded in agreement.

We all sat in silence the next 20 minutes before Ms. Vesuvius, dormant now, was escorted to one of the examining rooms. I followed to another room soon after.

No one takes more heat for asking people to wait than the pharmacist. I wonder how many people would be more patient in the pharmacy if they knew what goes on behind the counter. By that, I don't mean just telling them you're waiting for the prescribing doctor to OK a refill or you don't have enough stock of that drug or one pharmacist is out sick today or the computer is down.

Over time, when you can, in your way, tell *your* story. Tell people who you are and how you got where you are. Tell them what you do and what you'd like to do as part of a caring, changing profession.

With more knowledge, they'll come to appreciate what you do. And, they'll learn, as this impatient editor did, how to be more patient with their pharmacist.

Reprinted with permission from Drug Topics, © 1998; 142(16):14. Edited from the original.

AN ER PATIENT'S COMPLAINT

B. vön Koln Kleinmüntz

A heart patient who had been taken by ambulance to the same hospital ER with severe chest pain eight times in as many months, has now arrived again. A very friendly, but tired and shabby-looking intern, asks him, "what brings you here this morning?" Instead of responding with a cluster of symptoms, aches and pains as expected of him, the patient fires a volley of nonstop verbiage at the intern:

"Pay close attention. You are the first in a series of endless drowsy doctors-to-be who will surely be asking me the same questions. If I must repeat myself, I'll charge the lot of you tuition for pestering a person in pain; so assume the heavy responsibility of taking notes for the benefit of the rest of your crew lurking behind the desk sipping coffee ready to pounce upon me with identical queries.

"Here goes. I am 65 years old, and now have a chest pain of 3 on a scale of 1 to 10, with 10 being the most severe pain. When I called 911, my pain was at about 8 or 9 and I thought foolishly as it turns out but a better alternative to this—that it would do me in. But here I am. I've been here many times before, and my medical records are buried deep in the bowels of this hospital, and may be sent up before my insurance runs out, die—probably of boredom—or am discharged from the ER, and perhaps even from this hospital, whichever is later of course. In the interim of confusion, I inform you that I've had two coronary bypass procedures one in January of 1980, the other exactly seven years later neither of which was worth a damn. I am currently on this hospital's heart transplant list, and have been on it for eight months. I'm considering running for governor or becoming a ballplayer: They seem to have more luck procuring organs than I do. But why complain? That was Pennsylvania and California and this is Illinois. Such shenanigans would never happen here, at least not in Chicago, with its fine reputation for fair-play, honesty, and integrity.

"No, I don't smoke or drink—denies smoking and drinking in your language—but do have a family history of heart problems, my father having died of heart failure at the age of 86, and my mother at 82. My father was a heavy smoker, but not my mother. Go figure. I sleep on one pillow, not two, and my last chest pain was accompanied by some sweating—diaphoresis in your jargon—until the paramedics got the air conditioner going in the ambulance compartment.

"I have no shortness of breath, except when trying to explain my symptoms in the ER. My usual blood pressure is 100 over 60, but elevates somewhat during anginal pain and when badgered. Likewise, my pulse, usually at 60, rises to 85 when irritated by too many dumb questions. That's why I'm trying to anticipate as many of them now for surely if left to your discretion they'll be forthcoming soon.

"Don't worry, my crisis is over, and I won't die on your watch. Try not to lose the list of medications handed to you by my wife. If you do lose them, as did your colleagues on all prior eight occasions, make up a new list yourself. I'm on everything that ends in 'tec,' 'il,' 'xin,' and 'cardia.' I have no allergies, except to dumb questions. If you don't mind, I can now use a urinal. My lasix is beginning to act up. Oh, you don't do that, it's the nurse's job? Then why not let her ask me some dumb questions while you catch up on sleep?

"If you get a chance, please call, Dr. Samuels, spelled S-A-M-U-E-L-S, an attending cardiologist in this hospital who may, if you're lucky enough to locate him, fill you in on any details I may have omitted. You may have to place a long-distance call. The last I heard, he's in Tahiti and has no back-up on call. If you don't mind, I didn't sleep last night, and am tired as hell and would appreciate being left

Reprinted with permission from Journal of Irreproducible Results, © 1996; 41(1):7–8.

alone so that I can doze off before the nurses begin poking holes into my arms looking for veins that tend to roll and disappear before their very eyes; and before the X-Ray people arrive shouting 'X-Ray!' to let the nurses take cover to stay out of harm's way. In the meantime, get some coffee; you look awful, and your frayed jeans and rundown running shoes don't help. Is that supposed to be a tie around your neck? Does it light up? Isn't there some sort of dress code around here? Now go spread the word among your colleagues and tell them to stay the hell away from these shower curtains made to look like a room. Have a nice day."

SYPHILIS

Victor F. Tapson

You never know who you might meet,
No matter how polite and how sweet.
They won't have a sign,
"I've a Chancre on Mine,"
Or, "Check into Hotel Spirochete."

It always begins where exposed,
Your backside your front or your nose.
It later will spread,
To take your heart and your head,
Wreaking havoc wherever it goes.

The Treponemal Invader gets in,
And does all kinds of stuff to your skin,
Macules and scales,
Or mucous patch trails,
To your dermatologic chagrin.

They call it The Great Imitator.
A heart, nerve and bone/joint berator.
Your palms and your soles,
Are two of its goals,
It will get them *all* sooner or later.

If you had advanced lues today,
We could spot you from here to Bombay.
With your foot slappin' state,
And ataxic wide gait,
And your head that was bobbin' away.

If your lues is treated too slow,
You get tabes and joints of Charcot.
Even your brain,
Becomes gumma terrain,
Your pupils don't react or are slow.

The Jarisch-Herxheimer reaction,
Should actually give satisfaction.
Though you shake and you chill,
And you're violently ill,
It's caused by the bug's liquefaction.

So if your tendency is to transgress,
Look out for a spot that's painless,
Then think back to whom,
Imparted this gloom,
And find someone new to caress.

Without wearing the proper "attire,"
There's lots of things you could acquire.
But I would just chat,
And do no more than that,
Just sit and hold hands and admire.

Reprinted with permission from The Lancet, 1997; 350(9075):452, © by The Lancet Ltd.

WHAT TO DO WHEN YOU'RE SICK

Bill Ott

I like to think it was due to the 102-degree fever I was running, but on July 1, 1995, I concluded indubitably that Steven Seagall was my new favorite actor, his performance in *Under Siege* eclipsing even Jack Nicholson in *Chinatown* and Robert Mitchum in *Out of the Past*. During my illness, I also watched *The Unbearable Lightness of Being*, a film that I had managed to miss for years and was very excited to see. I hated it. Again, I'm assuming that my reaction had something to do with the unbearable lightheadedness of being I was experiencing at the time. Still, there seemed to be a pattern emerging, and I call it to your attention in hopes that you may be able to hasten your own recovery from your next illness. Here's the point: when your fever soars and your stomach turns, your taste changes. Not just your taste for food and drink, but also your taste for art and entertainment. Just as you wouldn't eat a five-course meal when you had the flu, so you need to dummy down your intake of film and literature. Art needs to be digested, too, after all. When your stomach requires softer food, your brain needs softer art. What follows is a list of qualities to avoid in films and reading material (providing reading is even an option) for those under the weather. I must add a caveat: my cure has the potential to become a disease of its own. I recently paid $7.50 to see the sequel to *Under Siege* and did so when I was perfectly healthy, my temperature holding securely at a constant 98.6 degrees. I thought it was a terrific movie and, as we speak, am considering moving on from Seagall to a full-scale investigation of the Jean-Claude Van Damme oeuvre.

Ambiguity: It is an established medical fact that human beings, when suffering from the flu, cannot tolerate ambiguity in any of its myriad forms. This means stay away—far away—from Henry James and any modern writer or filmmaker (be especially leery of foreign films) whose work suggests that reality may be this or it may be that or maybe it's all in how you see it. I'm a little dizzy right now just thinking about it. Also, be careful of children's books. Ambiguity has a way of sneaking into some of them, especially award winners. You've been warned.

Human relationships: You want to be alone when you're sick, right? So why would you want to read about or watch what happens to people when their emotions and hormones become inextricably intertwined with other people? Avoid Anne Tyler at all costs, and stay miles away from E. M. Forster. Don't connect.

Sex: Remember this simple rule: if you don't want to do it at the moment, you don't want to watch it being done. Or even hear how wonderful, how life-affirming, how transcendental, it can be. (Get thee to a nunnery, Lady Chatterley.)

Tricky Camera Angles: I dearly love film noir but not when I'm sick. Just imagine neon light flickering through half-closed Venetian blinds, and think how that might affect a queasy stomach. Farewell, my lovely noir. Another reminder: even brief contact with the phrase *mise en scene* is sure to cause a relapse.

Woody Allen: Woody Allen has made a brilliant career weighing and measuring all the psychic baggage—the fears and obsessions, the hypochondria, the guilt—that he has carried on his slender back all these years, but the last thing you want to hear when you're sick is a lot of witty moaning about the inevitability of death. And if that weren't enough, the word *nauseous* is uttered several times in every movie Woody Allen ever made. Case closed.

Reprinted with permission from Booklist, © 1995; 92(3):360. Edited from the original.

CONFESSIONS OF A STREET MEDIC

Jeff McBrayer

Dear Sirenhead: Forgive me, for I have sinned. If you will hear my confession it might save a life. I'm a fairly typical "dinosaur." Ever since I became a paramedic in 1985, my career has been my life. I used to look pretty stealth but when I hit 29, gravity kicked in. My aliases around the station include Buddha and Donut King. Now a not-too-stealthy 5'10", 210 lbs. (with gusts up to 225), I've got that perfect Homer Simpson gut that I can balance a Big Mac on while driving Code 3 through rush-hour traffic.

At home recently, watching the tube, I felt some chest pressure. Like the true health professional that I am, I ignored it. Four hours passed, and the chest pain persisted. As a bona fide American Heart Association ACLS instructor, I knew exactly what to do: I took more Tums. About an hour later I noticed I had a toothache. Strangely enough it was on both sides of my jaw. Not wanting to bother any of my colleagues for a ride, I popped two adult aspirins and drove to the station. Hooking myself up to the Lifepak 10, I immediately noticed sinus bradycardia and a rather large bundle branch block in Lead III. Because I've never run a marathon and my resting heart rate usually sits around 94, I was a little confused.

While discussing the merits of a modified chest lead (MCL 1) with another medic, he suddenly hit my mouth with two squirts of nitro spray. Within 30 seconds the chest pain was gone. Being the highly trained emergency responder that I am (read "Jeff is a dumb ass"), I drove myself to the ER.

The conversation at the ER went something like this: "Hey doc, how's it going? Looks like a busy shift. Oh yeah, could you run an EKG on me? I'm having a little chest pain that was relieved by nitro. . . ." Suddenly there was a flurry of activity. "Lie your ass down! IV and 02 over here! EKG stat! I need labs over here!"

"Yeah, doc, the chest pain is back. Gee, I feel sweaty. Yeah, doc, the nitro made it go away, but . . . transfer to CCU downtown? But I parked my car in police parking. Wow, triglycerides 505? But, doc, I'm taking Zocor for my cholesterol already. Family history? Well, my granddad died at 42 from an MI, but that was years before Zocor and stuff. . . ."

I wouldn't wish CCU on my worst enemy—not even my QA officer. Not because of the quality of care—but the sheer quantity of it: Nitro drip, heparin drip, blood draws every four hours, EKGs every four hours, automatic blood pressure checks every five minutes. Between the nitro headache (a chemically induced migraine to the 10th power-squared), the multiple IV sticks and the urinal—I'd take 10 shifts of system status management in downtown Baghdad any day!

It only gets worse when a cardiac surgeon you've known and respected for years looks down at you with that *"game face"* we all use when it's getting ugly, smiles and says: "Young fella, I think we better do a cath on you today."

I've treated hundreds of MI patients, delivered hundreds of patients to the cath lab. I told them all the same things the hospital staff told me: "We're doing everything we can to make you well and these folks will take great care of you." Now, when I speak to my patients, I can add, "I know how scared you must be because I know how scared I was."

I kept thinking, what will they find? Will they clear it with TPA or Streptokinase? Maybe a stint or a balloon angioplasty. God, please not a bypass. I'll never see my kid grow up if they bypass me at age 32. As I entered the cath lab, I remember thinking: "OK, no chest pain. I want to leave now. OK, I still have the chest pain but I don't give a s---. I want to leave now. They complete the quick prep in about five minutes, including Benadryl, (they give you that in case you're deathly allergic to the dye), a

---

Reprinted with permission from JEMS: Journal of Emergency Medical Services, © 1998; 23(5):96,98. Edited from the original.

quick shave of your entire right lower quadrant (and I do mean entire), a local anesthetic at the femoral site and 5 mg of Valium (because you're a medic and we feel sorry for you).

Let the games begin: I first felt the catheter somewhere in my subclavian, then again when they injected the dye into my coronary arteries. (That's the part when the elephant falls from the ceiling onto your chest.) Rinse and repeat, then onto the valve check, where about 72 gallons or so (my nearest approximation) of dye dumps into your heart. V-Tach was never so much fun! Then the Valium begins to kick in, and you're finished. Off to the recovery area to lie absolutely flat for seven hours (with a C-clamp on your crotch).

The verdict: "normal cardiac cath, rule out cardiac vasospasm vs. esophagitis." (Remember, dear colleagues, that nitro also relaxes the smooth muscle of the esophagus.) My upcoming upper GI series should reveal more. (Anyone who wants to share a barium shake—extra thick—feel free to give me a call.)

Have I gone to the land of sprouts and tofu? No, but now I don't even slow down to smell a Whopper combo meal. I traded Ben & Jerry's Chubby Hubby ice cream for Cherry Garcia frozen yogurt. Exercise? Yeah, I'm walking every day. (You try jogging after you've had a size 8 French catheter inserted in your right femoral artery.)

Am I gonna get philosophical, shouting *carpe diem*, quit my job, get in touch with my creative self? Hey, if it'll pay your rent, more power to you, but I'm running low on sick time and I'll go back on shift in another week. You'll find no mystery or moral to this story, just a realization that we are all mortal and have important responsibilities. No little "anti-cholesterol" pill and an aspirin a week will ever take the place of common sense, and it doesn't take that much effort to stay healthy. Thanks for lettin' me get another load off my chest.

Thanks for sharin', Donut King. I've worked with lots of guys like you—overweight and too busy to work out. At least you admit your mind was in vapor lock. You've probably lectured a hundred overweight cardiac time bombs about the need to access the EMS system as soon as any warning signs crop up. While I don't relish the thought of lugging your chubby butt down four flights of narrow stairs, call volume keeps me from getting laid off.

You know EMS can be a dog of a job and the Land of Cardiac Opportunity. When we're busy, nobody cares enough to allow us to take a decent rest break to relax and eat a healthy and uninterrupted meal. When we're not busy, our managers and dispatchers freak out and try to find assignments for us to handle. God forbid we have a half hour without the silver wheels turnin' and the cash register hummin'. This type of environment leads us to zip into a drive-through or some other grease pit and devour a rapid meal with a dose of high stress for dessert.

It doesn't end there at my full-time job. When I walk into my volunteer station, there's always somebody ordering a pizza, steak sandwiches, or chili dogs. Of course—to be sociable—I join in.

My point is that your weight isn't entirely your fault. You are a product of your environment. Stress makes you hungry as a bear, so it follows that a lot of EMS folks resemble bears. I envy some of my fire-medic pals because they have exercise rooms and excess hours (due to the traditional scheduling of crews to await unscheduled emergencies). They get to work off their fat while I have to sit my butt on a bucket seat 8 to 12 hours every shift. When my shift ends, I'm usually so wired I go out for a few beers and food to unwind. Then I go home and right to bed—only to repeat it all the next day.

Thanks for telling it like it is (was) and writing with such style. But, thanks especially for finally smartening up and working to shed the pounds. Your kid needs you and so do your co-workers. They may call you full-size nicknames, but you've earned them. They're probably just as concerned about your well-being as you are, but they'll never admit it to your face.

ONCOLOGISTS AND RADIOLOGISTS

Arthur W. Devermann

The following poem was written by a patient during his course of therapy:

Oncologists may treat all kinds of tumors by the score.

Radiologists see them as they're never seen before.

Sometimes they may shrink them with x-rays or lethal powers

Their treatment takes just seconds or minutes—but never hours.

It's miraculous how this science helps give brand new hope,

Renewing someone's zest for life and helping them to cope.

After higher education needed for this complex task,

They work at their professions and trust their treatments last

To restore Health and Happiness to all or just a few;

So if you need their services, they will do their best for you!

Reprinted with permission from Radiologic Technology, © 1985; 57(1):45.

MANAGING TO CARE

Managing to get paid for professional services has always been a tricky business. It never has been enough to just provide great patient care, somehow payment had to be exchanged between the patient and the provider. With the advent of managed care, a whole new set of rules must be strictly followed to survive any evolving scheme. Unseen hands are attempting to organize resources so that they are efficiently divided amongst competing parties. The real story here is that in the midst of revolutionary changes, ordinary health care professionals still manage to be attentive and caring.

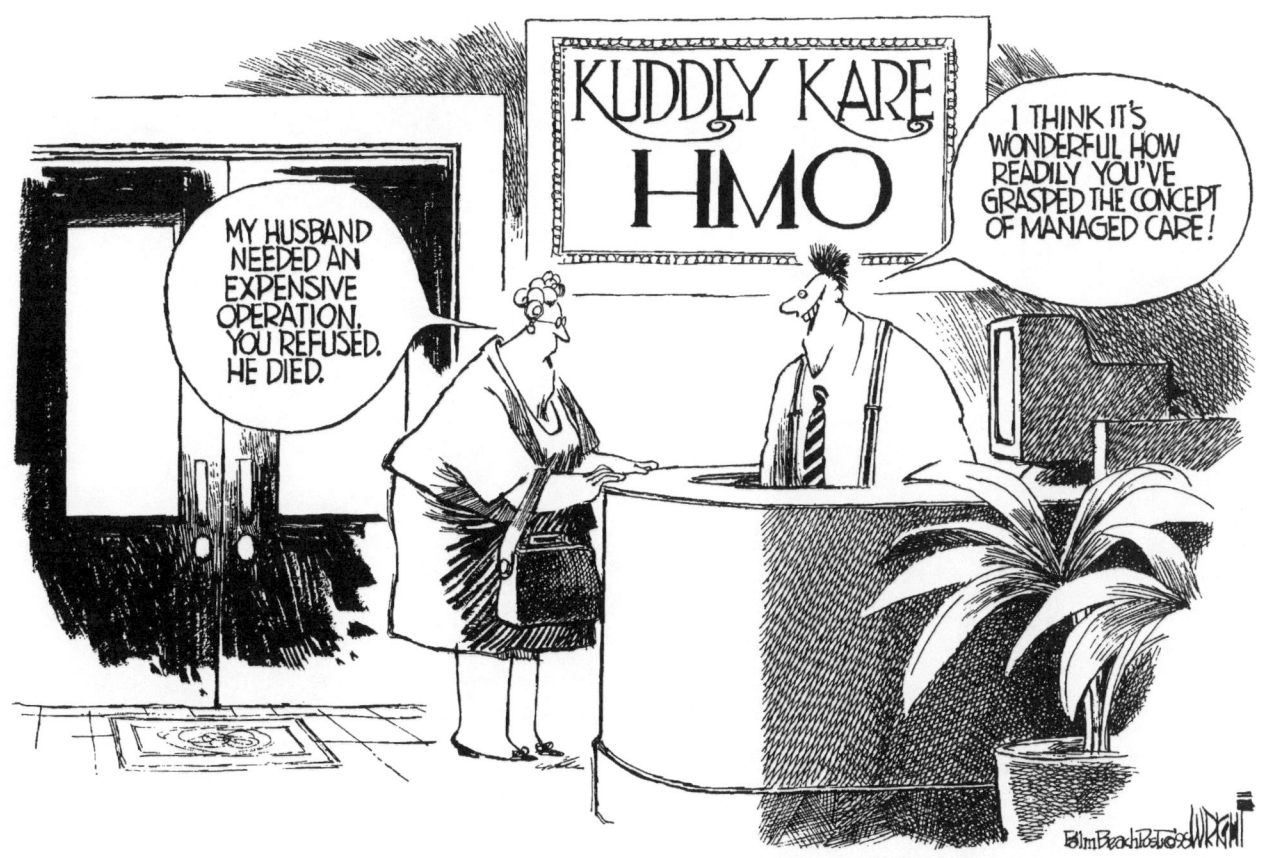

© Tribune Media Services, Inc. All Rights Reserved. Reprinted with permission.

FIRST, DO NO HARM
(PENDING PRIOR APPROVAL)

Alec Pruchnicki, MD

The scene: The office of the personnel director of a newly established health maintenance organization (HMO), who is interviewing a primary care physician.

HMO: Please come in and have a seat. I've been going over your CV and just have a few questions before I explain what we have to offer you. By the way, is Hippocrates your first name or last?

M.D.: I use only one name.

HMO: Your CV said you started your practice in Greece in about 400 B.C. We're normally not overly skeptical, but you don't really look your age.

M.D.: Well, I don't smoke, and I've always followed a strict Mediterranean diet. You know, lots of olive oil, fish, fresh fruits, and vegetables.

HMO: Oh, of course. Well, let's get down to business. Since our parent company, MiracleCo Insurance Underwriters, decided to set up an HMO, we here at Comprehensive Reliable Physician Care have been looking for qualified primary care physicians.

M.D.: Yes, I've heard your slogan: When you're covered by CRP Care, it's really a miracle.

HMO: I see you've completed all your foreign medical school exams, and you've gotten your license. Board certified?

M.D.: I was hoping I could qualify under the grandfather provision.

HMO: Okay, we can work on that. Our Public Relations—uh, I mean our Quality Assurance Department insists that we have all board-certified physicians. We usually don't look for academic types, but I notice that you've had a variety of publications in medicine, surgery, and other areas.

M.D.: I always tried to be well rounded and a generalist in my medical practice.

HMO: A generalist! Excellent, that's just the type we're looking for.

M.D.: I'm usually known for my oath. I thought everyone had at least heard of it during their training, even over here in the New World.

HMO: Well, I'm pretty well trained. I have a bachelor's in business finance and a master's in health care administration. But, it doesn't seem to ring a bell. What kind of oath is it?

M.D.: It's an oath of ethical behavior.

HMO: Oh. That explains it.

M.D.: There's a copy at the end of my CV.

HMO: Let's see. "I swear by Apollo the physician . . . blah, blah, blah . . . gods and goddesses. . . ." Sounds very classy.

M.D.: I tried my best.

HMO: ". . . to reckon him who taught me this Art equally dear to me as my parents. . . ."

M.D.: We had a high opinion of our teachers and treated them with respect.

HMO: Well, medical education doesn't fit into our program very well.

M.D.: Who will take care of medical education?

HMO: Who knows? Let's see, "I will impart a knowledge of the Art to my own sons, and those of my teachers . . . blah, blah . . . but to none others." Sounds pretty restrictive. Keeping down the supply helps control the marketplace. Are you sure you never took business administration yourself?

M.D.: No, we just learned as we went along.

HMO: We have women doctors now, too.

M.D.: I can live with that.

HMO: "I will give no deadly medicine to anyone if asked, nor suggest any such counsel. . . ." So you had problems with the euthanasia debate back then?

M.D.: Quite a bit, that's why it's in the oath. If we didn't control it, before long people could be using it for convenience or to save money on medical costs for their elderly and frail.

Reprinted with permission from New England Journal of Medicine, 337(22), Nov 27, 1997:1627–1628. Copyright © 1997, Massachusetts Medical Society. All rights reserved.

HMO: Uh, yeah, we couldn't have that. Where were we? "I will not give to a woman a pessary to produce abortion." Well, we have physicians who will provide these services if requested, but I can certainly see why you would want to avoid controversy.

M.D.: I put it in out of conviction, not to avoid contro—

HMO: Whatever. "I will not cut persons laboring under the stone, but will leave this to be done by men who are practitioners of this work." So, you don't like surgical procedures. Great! "I . . . will abstain from every voluntary act of mischief and corruption; and, further from the seduction of females or males, of freemen and slaves." I like this part about females and males, very politically correct. But, this part about slaves—

M.D.: It was written a long time ago. We can lose the "slave" part.

HMO: Okay. "Whatever, in connection with my professional service, or not in connection with it, I see or hear, in the life of men, which ought not to be spoken of abroad, I will not divulge, as reckoning that all such should be kept secret." Well, so signing a gag clause and not giving out confidential information wouldn't bother you?

M.D.: Of course not. Confidentiality about my patients' medical conditions is essential to my medical ethics.

HMO: Uh, that's not exactly what I had in mind. Your patients' records may be available to us or other insurers, physicians, maybe even employers.

M.D.: That seems pretty unethical to me. So, what do you keep confidential?

HMO: Mostly financial agreements between the physicians, such as you, and the HMO. Also, we prefer that you do not tell the patients about medical procedures that are not covered by their policies. We believe in that old expression, "First, do no harm." Maybe you've heard of it?

M.D.: Yes, I've heard of it. But it was used to warn against doing medical harm to the patients, not financial harm to the insurance company. How will we be able to counsel the many sick and frail patients who come to us?

HMO: Many sick and frail patients? Let me explain how we work here at CRP Care. Most of our patients enroll through their employers, so they are usually fairly healthy. The surest way to make money in this business is to avoid sick people as much as possible and seek out healthy ones.

M.D.: How do I know which procedures are covered?

HMO: You contact us ahead of time for major procedures, tests, consultations, hospitalizations, and such, and we approve or deny payment depending on the criteria we have set up.

M.D.: That's quite a list of items. Doesn't it bother you to be second-guessing medical decisions?

HMO: Oh, we never second-guess medical decisions. After all, we're an insurance company; we don't practice medicine. We just tell you what we'll pay for. You and the patient can decide on anything you want. I know it's a subtle distinction, but it's very important to our control of expenses.

M.D.: While not actually taking the blame if anything goes wrong. Very ingenious. Back in Greece we had a group of philosophers called the Sophists. You would like them.

HMO: Well, our legal department is still hiring. Send them around. But we don't expect you to take risks for nothing. We have a wide range of financial bonuses if you come in under budget.

M.D.: And if I'm over budget?

HMO: Well, there are financial penalties if you exceed your budget. But I'm sure a person with your experience will know how to run a practice within guidelines.

M.D.: Maybe experience is the key. This system is new. As time goes on, the physicians and other providers will explain things to the administrators and financial people and set things straight.

HMO: Uh, I've got some more bad news for you, Dr. H. It's the financial and business people who run things around here, not the physicians or anyone else. Don't hold your breath waiting for them to come around asking for advice.

M.D.: So it won't get any better?

HMO: Better! Once all the doctors and patients are signed up who can be signed up, it will probably get a lot worse. Some doctors may even find themselves in an oversupply status.

M.D.: You mean unemployed.

HMO: Yes, unemployed. But remember, since we don't provide for medical education, the supply of physicians will eventually shrink to meet our budgets.

M.D.: Wonderful. So, let me see now. We tend to the healthy and avoid the sick. We are rewarded for providing the least care and penalized for providing the most care. This is in a medical system that has minimal concern for ethics, hides information from the patients, and is run by financial people instead of doctors, nurses, or anyone else who cares for the patients.

HMO: Now you've got it, Dr. H. See how easy it is to understand? And you continue to be an independent contractor, especially in terms of risk, since we—

M.D.: I know, I know, you don't practice medicine. Well, my friends warned me about all this, but I had to hear it for myself. I'm sorry, but I don't think I can practice medicine in this system.

HMO: All the other HMOs are about the same. If you don't sign up now, you may be locked out.

M.D.: Maybe I've been in practice long enough. Over the years I've invested in some olive groves back in Greece. I could probably do all right just with them. "Bailing out" is the expression, right?

HMO: I'm afraid so. It's too bad. A person with your experience would be a real asset to CRP Care, in spite of that ethical stuff. Are you sure I can't get you to reconsider?

M.D.: I'm sure. Sorry for wasting your time, but I was hoping there would be some way to do this.

HMO: Well, Dr. H., let me make one suggestion—though I don't know why I'm saying this, since it can't possibly profit CRP Care. Before you go home to Greece, stop off in Canada.

M.D.: Thank you for the advice.

HMO: Well, let me see you to the door, Dr. H. I hope everything works out all right, and don't forget that side trip. Goodbye now. Okay, next applicant. Dr. Maimonides? Please come in.

BREAST REDUCTION AD ABSURDUM

Robert M. Goldwyn, MD

I. Trickham and U. Killum, co-founders of Total Care, the fastest growing Health Maintenance Organization in America, were in an emergency session.

"Two got through," Trickham said mournfully. "I can't believe it, but in Peoria we actually had to pay for two women's breast reductions."

"You mean, they met our criteria?" Killum asked in wonderment.

"Yup. They were twins with the ideal height and weight according to our chart: 4'2", 82 lbs, with a bra size of 48DDD. Each of them had acute and chronic pain of her back, neck, and shoulders, with numbness in her hands and rashes under her breasts. Each had documented 102 visits with an orthopedic surgeon and 75 with a chiropractor. Each of them had been 4 years in casts and back supports, with photographic proof!"

"Astounding, almost impossible," Killum murmured, his head in his hands. "Dear Lord, what next?"

"Well, when you think of it, only two women out of 350,000 over 4 years."

"But, even so. Once something like this happens, the floodgates are open. We might have to pay for three more over the next 40 years. This will kill us. Just when we thought we had a fail-safe program. Remember we paid that statistician $20,000 to come up with stringent criteria. He is a phony."

"Don't be so hard on him. He tried his best. I'm a step ahead of you," replied Trickham with a grin. "I already called Professor Goodstats. Let me read his letter."

'Dear Mr. Trickham:

'Although I enjoy hearing from you, I was appalled, nevertheless, by your startling news. I can

---

Reprinted with permission from Plastic and Reconstructive Surgery, © 1998; 102(1):246.

understand your anger and disappointment that your insurance company had to honor commitments to these two women. The question now is, what steps can we take to see that this situation never again arises?

'I have concluded that the requirements that I once proposed and you enacted cannot now be strengthened or made more prohibitive with regard to the patient. But there is a way out. Because of the concept of 'coupling'—something that I originated—not only must the patient meet certain requirements, but the surgeon also. The reality is that both the patient and the doctor are in a relationship, and neither is exempt in this duality. What I most strongly recommend, therefore, as additional criteria for coverage, is that the birthdate of the surgeon and his or her height and weight be identical to the birthdate and the height and weight of the patient. With these additional requirements, I can assure you that never again will Total Care have to cover reduction mammaplasty.

'If I may be so bold as to paraphrase our beloved Abraham Lincoln, you can cover some of the people all of the time and all of the people some of the time, but not all of the people all of the time and in the instance of Total Care, none of the people any of the time! . . .'"

Killum rises, his face beaming.

"Trickham, you and Goodstats have restored my faith in corporate America. I always said that no bottom-line thinking can ever be below the belt."

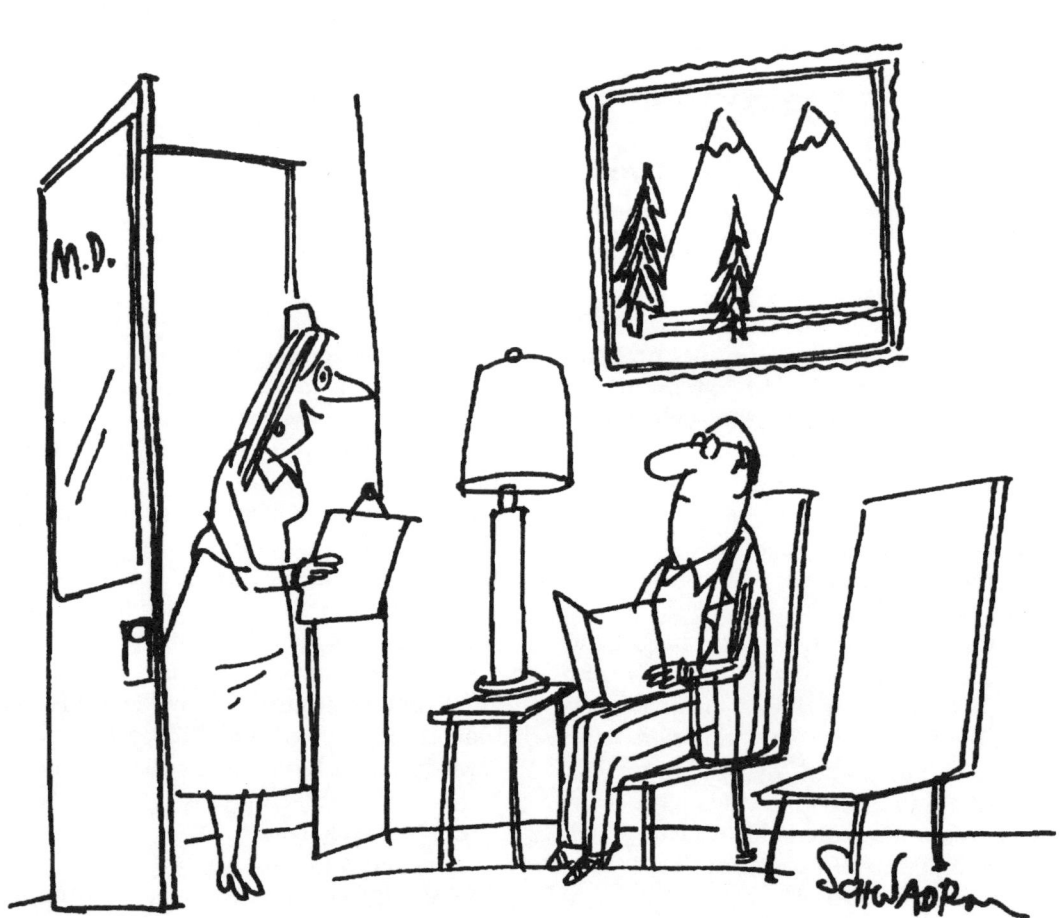

"We're taking a poll. Would you prefer computerized billing and diagnosis by a human, or human billing and computerized diagnosis?"

© 1998 Medical Economics.

UP TO YOUR WAIST IN ALLIGATORS?

Barbara Penn

For the second time in my life as an occupational therapist, I have resigned my post due to my inability to see eye to eye with the Government of the day which has, in my view, been "economical with the truth."

All politicians would have us believe that they are concerned about the environment. In the last year alone, the National Health Service must take responsibility for destroying at least one rain forest and increasing pollution in the atmosphere, as we all disappeared under a mountain of paper and burned the midnight oil. The result of this labour was the production of contracts, inches thick, and now probably gathering dust on shelves all over the country. The aim of the exercise . . . to improve the quality of the Health Service and to offer patients increased choice in health care.

The incidence of ill-health rises with age and has a close association with poverty and social class. Do people falling into these categories truly have a choice? What about people like me, living on an island that has a high percentage of unemployment and a large elderly population? I wonder whether districts will readily agree to be parted from their cash to foot the cross-boundary charges if we all opt to exercise our choice?

And what about this nebulous term, quality? Those of you familiar with *Zen and the Art of Motorcycle Maintenance* will understand the sanity-threatening struggle of one man to define and live a life of quality.

How is it that quality is always inextricably linked with finance? Whilst we have all been beavering away over the last 12 months, the accountants have cloned. We all know that money to pay for the Health Service is not inexhaustible, but I wonder when the armed services will begin to hold jumble sales to buy armaments?

The Health Service has become the "health care industry" and whether we like or accept this term is of no importance to the politicians. The difficulty faced by all health services now that we are a business venture is to calculate how best to capture accurate data describing the treatment of a patient whilst maintaining quality of care and how to place a realistic cost on the treatment delivered.

In the USA, cost is based on the use of Diagnostically Related Groups and a version of this method is likely to be used in this country. The interesting thing about the use of this method is that DRGs were developed as a means of improving the quality of treatment for patients and were later taken up by accountants as a means of costing that same commodity. By applying this model to health care, it becomes possible to equate the industrial terms of product selection, quality control and cost accounting to the health care sector. The danger is that by changing the emphasis from one of improving quality to one of controlling costs, sight is lost of the original objective. Rather like the story of the man who found himself up to his waist in water and surrounded by alligators. He was so taken with saving his own life that he lost sight of his original objective . . . which was to drain the swamp.

Reprinted with permission from British Journal of Occupational Therapy, © 1991; 54(7):243.

PHARMACY-BUZZWORD BINGO

Bruce A. Mueller, PharmD, FCCP
Bruce C. Carlstedt, PhD

Recently, we became aware of a "buzzword bingo card" designed to help a person not fall asleep during business meetings. The squares in this Dilbert-esque game contained business lingo, such as "gap analysis," "the big picture," "the bottom line," "results-driven," and "shift your paradigm." Indeed, there is a Web site dedicated to this game: http://www.buzzwordbingo.com.

After using a printout of the bingo card at one of our own meetings, we decided that a card could be made specifically for pharmacy meetings. We propose a pharmacy-buzzword bingo game for use during any pharmacy-related meeting. The user would simply holler "Bingo!" when he or she has crossed off five boxes lined up on a diagonal, row, or column, or the four boxes in the outer corners.

An example of a pharmacy-buzzword bingo card appears below. As we put this project together, we quickly realized that there are more pharmacy buzzwords than can fit on a single bingo card. Thus, we have included extra words that can be used to personalize a bingo card. When you make these cards, we request only that "pharmaceutical care" be placed in the center, as it has become the mother of all buzzwords.

Disclaimer: We will not be held responsible for demotions, pay cuts, or unemployment deriving from the use of pharmacy-buzzword bingo.

Documentation	Intervention	Narrow Therapeutic Index	Continuity of Care	Evidence-Based
Patient Outcomes	Product-Centered	Internet Pharmacy	Self-Care	"Pharmaco-" as a prefix
Most-Trusted Professional	Cognitive Service	Pharmaceutical Care	Pharmacy is at the Crossroads	Lick, Stick, Count, and Pour
In the Basement	Drug Misadventure	Fee-for-Service	On the Floors	All-Pharm.D.
Pharmacist Certification	Disease State Management	Cost-effective	Pharmacist-Run	Patient-Focused

Sample bingo card. Additional terms for personalized bingo cards include the following: Discharge Counseling, Women in Pharmacy, Clinical Pharmacy, Pharmacotherapeutic, Translational Research, Empower the Patient, Value-Added, Medication-Use System, Pharmacoeconomic, Binding Sites, Central Pharmacy, Decentralized Pharmacy, Baker Cells, Computerized Record, Complementary & Alternative Medicine, Certificate Program, Patient Education, Noncompliance, www.anything, and Continuing Competence.

Reprinted with permission from American Journal of Health-System Pharmacy, © 1999; 56(23):2464.

A MODEST PROPOSAL

A Satirical Look at Managed Care
James F. Lally, MD

Jonathan Swift's grim, satirical essay *A Modest Proposal*, which to this day still generates controversy, suggested that the solution to the seemingly eternal problem of the poor in Ireland is to feed the entrails of the poor children to the rich.

Both parties of this unique, albeit indecorous, arrangement benefit; the rich pay the parents for the children and the rich in turn are well fed. Such controversial ideas that are well beyond the boundaries of conventional thinking, I believe, are what is needed to deal boldly and aggressively with the onslaught of managed care.

Part of the implied agenda for managed care is to reduce the future supply of physicians. Eli Ginzberg agrees with other medical leaders that there is a surplus of medical students and residents in training. He also points out that organized medicine and the federal government have done little more than recognize that there may be a problem. But, Ginzberg and other medical pundits are not thinking or approaching the problem in a shrewd, discerning, Swiftian manner. Trying to restrict the number of physicians may not solve the problem; increasing the number of potential patients for all those newly-minted physicians will. Now that you've refocused your thinking and changed your ethos, an array of novel, but controversial, solutions will seem obvious.

Since the Supreme Court's landmark decision in Roe v. Wade in 1973, it has been estimated that over 30 million abortions have been performed in the United States. Try to think of this not as 30 million abortions but rather as 30 million potential patients that have been lost to medicine. Those numbers suggest that we could have been increasing the supply of obstetricians and pediatricians, not decreasing them. Organized medicine and individual practitioners may want to rethink their ideas about abortion when they realize that every abortion results in one lost future patient.

Likewise, at the other end of life, euthanasia and assisted suicide, although they do not account for a great number of early deaths in this country, should be discouraged as they decrease the potential number of patients that our fledgling physicians could care for.

It has been charged that tobacco addiction remains one of the foremost causes of premature death in this country. Indeed, the acrimonious debate over the role of tobacco as the cause of disease has spawned the term "tobacco wars." But smokers want their right of free choice and there are those who think it is a politically dangerous precedent to limit the rights of others when it does not clearly obstruct their own right to free expression. In addition, it has been forcefully argued that tobacco farmers have a right to make a living. There is also a forgotten political spin-off from treating patients with tobacco addiction in their 40s and 50s; the rest of society will not have to pay their social security benefits except for those few heavy smokers that live beyond their mid 60s.

All of the frenetic national efforts at wellness and public health preventive measures seem laudatory but in reality they limit the number of potential patients for physicians of the 21st century.

Congress should immediately follow Germany's progressive attitude of allowing unrestricted speed on the autobahn and legislate unlimited speed on interstate highways. This will further justify the need for those Level 1 trauma centers that are so expensive to support and maintain and, as an added benefit, it will strengthen training programs in emergency care and trauma.

In your own practice, and as an informed citizen, make every effort to support those political programs, such as immigration and open borders, that will increase the population. Sure, those policies

Reprinted with permission from Delaware Medical Journal, © 1998; 70(10):441–442.

will increase the rolls of welfare recipients, but America can probably easily feed and house a billion people. Doesn't one of our larger agriculture conglomerates advertise that they are the "supermarket to the world?"

Liberalize your attitude about illicit drugs and encourage efforts to legalize marijuana. Also, petition your local legislator to lower the legal age for drinking.

The list could go on, but you get the point and I'm sure you could offer some of your own solutions. Swift was right, sometimes the solution to complex, apparently unsolvable problems is right in front of us—we just have to look for it.

I'VE BECOME THE PERFECT HMO PROVIDER!

Stanley J. Savinese, DO

Recently, I received my worst evaluation ever from one of the biggest HMOs in my area. According to the appraisers, my medical care had declined sharply since my last report card. This sort of news always strikes terror in the heart of us type-A i-dotters and t-crossers. And never mind that the displeased HMO had already cut my salary 20 percent.

How, I wondered, had I fallen so far into the abyss of poor patient management? Did I fail to screen for high cholesterol in 21-year-old women? Did I neglect to advise 28-year-old men seeking treatment for tennis elbow to have a prostate exam? Did I overlook an opportunity to document explicit sexual histories of elderly dowagers? Did I forget to do testicular checks on 8-year-old boys when their moms brought them in with the sniffles?

No, no, no, and no! My HMO had detected similar oversights during previous quality reviews, but I'd rectified them. Hey, I don't just do what's good for my patients, I do what my betters tell me. So where had I gone wrong this time?

The answer: I'd failed to document in my charts that I'd told several patients to wear bicycle helmets and install smoke detectors.

At first I envisioned myself going postal at the HMO's headquarters. But then I realized something: *I was guilty!* No question, they had me cold.

So, to avoid future lapses in preventive care, I developed a questionnaire for my patient's charts that reviews and forbids any behavior that might prove expensive for the HMO. For instance, why stop with bicycle helmets? Shouldn't it be the doctor's job to ensure that patients wear proper headgear in all situations? Of course. I now remind everyone in my care to wear rain hats in the rain, sun hats in the sun, and those little visors when playing poker.

My newly revised medical charts not only reflect in-depth personal probings, unending health screenings, vaccination and re-vaccination for all preventable diseases, but now I can honestly say that I've removed completely the need for my patients to have a mother, grandmother, or clergyman. In fact, they don't even need a whit of common sense.

The quality of my medical care has soared to new heights now that, in addition to being available to my patients 24 hours a day, 365 days per year, I have taken control of their lives and eliminated any possible predisposition they may have had to do anything that might jeopardize the HMO's bottom line.

Once you've reviewed my patient questionnaire (see next page), you'll want to include it in all of your charts. When this document appears in every patient record in the country, perhaps we can return to our secondary jobs: to alleviate suffering.

Copyright © 1998 by Medical Economics. Reprinted by permission from Medical Economics Magazine; 75(3):147–148.

DR. SAVINESE'S SAVE-MONEY-FOR-THE-HMO PATIENT QUESTIONNAIRE

Dear Patient:

The purpose of this questionnaire is to find out what you're doing and make you stop. The correct answers are indicated below.

1. *Do you drink, smoke, take drugs, have sex, drive faster than the speed limit, avoid seat belts, walk barefoot, eat candy, or go outside with wet hair?*
   A. I used to go barefoot, but stopped.
   B. I would never consider doing any of those things, ever.

2. *Do you report routinely to your family doctor for testing to detect any possible early-stage disease, and request embarrassing, invasive exams, even when your complaint is a sore toe? Also, do you refuse to visit specialists, have X-rays, and obtain prescriptions?*
   A. A doctor once prescribed penicillin for me, but now I'm allergic to it.
   B. Insurance companies have suffered enough. I'd never dream of costing them money.

3. *Do you wear proper headgear in all situations; never leave home without mittens, scarf, galoshes, and umbrella; associate with only nice people; get proper rest; and avoid watching violent TV shows?*
   A. One of my galoshes has a hole in it.
   B. Yes, and thanks for asking.

4. *Does your diet consist exclusively of green, leafy vegetables (not including tobacco), whole grains, legumes, eight glasses of pure mountain spring water per day, and tofu?*
   A. I used to eat fish, but gave it up.
   B. Yes. We are what we eat. I'm an organic farmer near Boston.

5. *Do you engage in tendon-sparing, low-impact aerobic exercise at least five hours per week, bathe twice daily, avoid buildings without windows, and live in a germ- and allergen-free plastic bubble?*
   A. One week I exercised for only four hours.
   B. Yes. The last speck of pollen was just removed from my environment.

6. *Do you promise to engage in only the healthiest practices imaginable in every facet of your life, every second of every day, so long as you shall live?*
   A. I want to have fun, so I'm willing to pay extra for my insurance premium.
   B. I do.

The correct answer to each question is B. If you have a perfect score, your HMO and I hereby deem you a worthwhile and healthy person.

If you've chosen other answers for any reason, you're an incorrigible lout and probably have scurvy. You must improve your behavior to ensure good health and avoid costly expenditures by your insurance company.

A POP QUIZ

Mary Grayson

It's time for a little pop quiz to test your knowledge of health care management issues. Don't be frightened. I'm sure you'll do just fine. So just grab a pencil, squeeze that Bic, or juice up the old Mont Blanc. Here we go!

1. **What's a sure sign that you're in really big trouble?**
   a. There's a bunch of FBI guys sitting in your office waiting to see you.
   b. The IRS keeps calling.
   c. Your mother stops talking to you.
   (c. That's right. No one is more important than Mom.)

2. **Is upcoding permissible?**
   a. Yes.
   b. No.
   c. Maybe.
   (c. But check your manual. See page 15,782 under rule No. 10,569,321.56.)

3. **To cut operating expenses, you should:**
   a. Fire the first person you see in the hallway.
   b. Outsource everything.
   c. Water down the Jell-O.
   (a. If he's not in his office, it's obvious that he's a time-waster. You can't possibly water down the Jell-O. Patient satisfaction will plummet. The earth will stop spinning, and the world will come to an end.)

4. **What should you tell the top surgeon who wants you to buy the latest Bitsy Big-Boy Boomeroo?**
   a. If the guy is over 45, tell him that the Health Planning Act has just been reinstated. Say that you'll really try your best, but it will probably take years.
   b. If he's under 45, tell him that all of the managed care companies have banded together and refuse to pay for Bitsy Big-Boy Boomeroo procedures.
   c. Lunge across the desk and choke him until he loses consciousness.
   (c. It's always best to take decisive action. And that's the last you'll ever see of that troublemaker, by golly.)

5. **What's the best answer to give pesky trustees who ask why almost everyone admitted to the hospital dies?**
   a. Act surprised and say you'll get right on it.
   b. Blame materials management.
   c. Be assertive: Blame them. After all, they're ultimately responsible for quality.
   (b. Say that materials management has been buying the wrong supplies, but the situation has been corrected.)

6. **What should you do when the managed care negotiator says that you must lower prices or get dropped?**
   a. If you're retiring the next day, say no.
   b. If you can't retire, say you'll think about it.
   c. Lunge across the desk and choke him until he loses consciousness.
   (c. Don't you wish.)

7. **What's the point of this column?**
   a. There isn't one.
   b. It's time to take a vacation.
   c. Everyone in health care should lighten up and have some fun.
   (All of the above!)

Reprinted from *Hospitals & Health Networks*, Vol. 71, No. 16, by permission, August 20, 1997. Copyright 1997, by Health Forum, Inc.

ADVENTURES IN THE PA TRADE

David Wolman, PA-C

In 1991 I graduated from a physician assistant program in a diverse class. The average age was 30 something, so unless we had been in the jury pool for a celebrity murder trial, *there had been life before PA school.*

In fact, I had been a novelist, a muralist, and an organic farmer. I had produced plays. And I had been an emergency medical technician (EMT) on a volunteer ambulance squad in rural New York, where the average run required at least one stop to fill the tank.

What I had *not* been was a college student for 17 years. So I tuned myself up with a few science courses and found that I could do quite well in PA school at an advanced age (39). But after I passed the boards and began my job hunt, I became fearful of being pegged a weird, middle-aged, neurotic escapee from the Walter Mitty Home for the Diversely Experienced.

It Begins

On my first job interview, a dour chief of general surgery confirmed my worst fear. He looked at my resumé and asked why someone with multiple degrees and a varied background wanted to be a PA.

"I believe," I said, "that all of this complements my skills as a physician extender." He looked at me as though "physician extender" were synonymous with "Tuna Helper."

Eventually, I was hired by a colorectal surgeon who had never employed a PA. He was creative, too: He painted abstract intestines that hung on the walls of his waiting room.

And he didn't have to bother with HMOs, PPOs, or Cheerios. He was strictly SRO, with while-you-wait wallet biopsies. His surgical skills came so well recommended that he considered interaction with his patients unnecessary. He never bothered to introduce me to any of his helpless, recumbent patients before he probed, like Captain Nemo with a fiberoptic scope, the inner depths of their haustra (later immortalized in acrylic on canvas).

I Move On

I noticed an ad for "house officer" at a major pediatric rehab hospital. "Treatment teams" were mentioned. Maybe there would be intramurals?

I got the job. "Treatment teams" turned out to be pig Latin for "procrastination brigades." In endless meetings, everyone marked out their territory and took action at the speed of a glacier. I loved the kids, but I never got to see them. They were obscured by incomprehensible bureaucracy—a syrupy mixture of hospital documentation, utilization review, multiple insurance mania, city and state regulation, overworked and ineffectual child protection services, and federal gobbledygook.

Yet all was not lost. I now knew which pens cut best through five carbons.

I Forge Ahead

I took a job with an austere, entrepreneurial, West Philadelphia physician in an impoverished, medically underserved neighborhood. He had the right multicultural and alternative lifestyle posters on his walls, but had come to accept his patients as "capitated lives." (That sounded like Robespierre at work in a health care Reign of Terror.) Never fear, change is good, he told me, as long as we know the right ICD-9-CM codes.

The office received bonuses from managed care groups for not referring to specialists ("utilization points") and for not closing to new patients. This made for a swelling practice that provided every cure one can imagine except pedicures.

Reprinted with permission from Journal of the American Academy of Physician Assistants, © 1995; 8(9):21,25,28.

When we did refer (drawing the line at transplanting hearts), we had to know our details—such as which nicotine patch was reimbursable by which managed care group on a particular day. Reimbursements were placed in the hands of a cadre of Generation X front-office workers who were compensated with free nose piercings.

Quarterly, the boss presented us with color-coded pie charts that showed how many patients we had seen, and on which we were labeled "producers." I caught on early to a basic principle: In theory, the more patients I saw, the more money I would make.

Truth is, patients in this practice of the future were widgets, not human beings. Producers weren't much better off; our antennae were weighted down with pollen. Meanwhile, profit-sharing checks were based on an arcane formula known only to the physician and paid out on a schedule as reliable as space shuttle launch times.

Most patients were poor. I was instructed to spend as little time as possible with elderly indigents who had "the wrong kind of insurance."

The real motive of this masquerading self-righteous businessman was *revenge* against what he saw as a system imposed unfairly—revenge in the form of big bucks and deferential employees. If he could use managed care, the poor, and naive PAs to reach these goals, well, that was in keeping with the American way of medicine and business.

Perhaps this is why the chief executive officer of U.S. Healthcare has a salary in the millions while millions in the U.S. have no health care.

Later, I learned, this sweatshop was gobbled up by a hungry provider network. Patients were sent a form letter assuring them of continuity of indifference.

My consolation? I can insert Norplant capsules with my eyes closed.

I Quit

Was I suffering from an employment disorder? I was reassured by the director of my PA program that it was common for graduates to change jobs frequently the first few years out.

I went back to the drawing board and reassessed my employment strategy. I read novels, took walks in the state park, and reflected on the simple, visceral job of having helped people as an EMT.

An Itinerant and Happy PA

The result of my meditation was that I found a job in a family practice in rural West Chester, PA, 2 days a week, with a scrupulous physician—where, despite the constraints of managed care, patients are treated well. And I took a second job in an emergency room in Delaware 2 days a week, with an employer who respects employees. Here, my former preceptor supervises a band of funny, congenial PAs who refuse to become cynical.

I also lecture at my PA alma mater. Teaching reacquainted me with the fact that medicine is fascinating and that the human body is beautiful, not bureaucratic.

But Times Are Troubled

Today, there is a confusing smorgasbord of job choices and many troubling moral ambiguities for PAs. Managed care can be mangled care. It took me 4 years and 5 jobs to realize that amenable colleagues and good relationships with my patients are more important than fancy jargon and the bells and whistles hawked in a job description.

Caring for the ill has always been something between a science and a calling, between a profession and a charitable endeavor. Until we get the mix right—under a system of universal coverage or pyramidal cost shifting—we may suffer because of our ambivalence.

Today, insurance companies and managed care networks are buying up practices to achieve, like Disney and Microsoft, "vertical integration"—which means that they aim to control the patients, the physicians, the PAs, the hospitals, and the drug companies. In the end, they may dictate care based on corporate earnings—the way that entertainment networks are managed by former agents and entrepreneurs, not by the creative people who provide the talent and the products.

And in the offing are more satellite urgent-care centers, fast-foodlike drive-throughs where medicine can be dispensed like a Happy Meal.

My Idea of Indemnity

I consider myself flexible and progressive—I think I had the first Macintosh computer ever built. But I refuse to give up the principles that brought me into the world of healing because of lobby-dominated politics or the exigencies of NASDAQ.

I feel that I owe my patients more than seeing four of them an hour, and the PA profession more than a quota of CME credits. I have a personal responsibility to continue becoming an ethical healer and a well-rounded human being, which is tantamount to keeping my resumé as weird as possible.

A HEALTHCARE PARABLE

William R. Pentecost, NREMT-P

The morning clouds were as gloomy as his mind. When Steve Custer awoke that morning, his heart sank. He recalled how just last evening he'd received the bad news—he was included in the lawsuit against the outfielders of the Portland Penguins. He'd worked so hard and studied so long to become a professional baseball player, and did everything in his power to catch that fly ball. Now, just because he had missed it by 2 inches, they were all being sued by the fans.

"Sometimes I wonder if it's really worth it," he mused. "All those years of college, prebaseball school, and then 4 years of an internship followed by 2 more years as a resident player—all for a lousy $200,000!" He then recalled how he'd opened the letter informing him that his malcatch insurance was being increased by one-third again, for the second time in 3 years, while painfully aware that the malpass and malcatch insurance for professional football players had tripled during the same time period. He began to feel guilty about complaining, realizing that at least baseball players were still making enough to afford a new car every 2 years.

The harsh ringing of the phone interrupted his thoughts. He picked up the receiver. "What are you going to do about it?" said the voice at the other end. It was his best friend, Jerry Hampton, the team's prized pitcher. "I thought I had it bad, but now..." Jerry's voice trailed off. "I sure wish I knew—maybe we could form a union, too. Then we could go on strike for a month and get free-agency, too," replied Steve. "Those doctors sure have it made, don't they?" he remarked.

"Yeah, do they ever—charging a million apiece for a lousy appendectomy, $10 million for a liver transplant—and not even having to pay a cent for malpractice or anything!" said Jerry.

"And the sponsors paying $2 million for a 30-second stint on the commercials. Who wants to watch a heart/lung transplant on the Super Surge once a year anyway?" growled Steve.

"Then they have all those perks, like news briefs, appearances in Rolaids and Alka-Seltzer commercials... and those nurses—look at them. They charge a half a million for an appearance on *The Late Show* and $2 million for a week's worth of home visits!

"And those paramedics—wow! They charged my father-in-law $10,000 just for a ride to the hospital when he had a stomach problem! Man, it makes my blood boil!" lamented Jerry.

"And to think they get away with all those times they mess up—man, if I only batted .900, or caught only 95% of the fly balls that come my way, I would be in the poor house!" moaned Steve.

"Last week, a visiting nurse came to visit my mother-in-law. She tried twice to insert a Foley and three times to start an IV before she got that right, and the reporters waiting to interview her trampled down all our azalea bushes!" Jerry retorted.

Steve agreed: "Wow, I just don't think it's right! Maybe someday society will wake up to the true values in life!"

Reprinted with permission from Emergency Medical Services, ©1997; 26(6):12,14. Edited from the original.

IN THE PUSH TO EXPLORE NEW FRONTIERS

Lynn Wagner

In the push to explore new frontiers, we can't afford to forget the more mundane challenges facing us.

So, it has come to this: We can clone a sheep but can't figure out a rational way to finance long-term care.

Obviously, these two things have absolutely nothing to do with each other. But stunning scientific breakthroughs that on the surface have little or nothing to do with the rhythms of daily life invite such juxtapositioning. A good example is the question posed decades ago, "How is it we can put a man on the moon but can't find a cure for the common cold?"

Before Neil Armstrong and Buzz Aldrin took that historic step for mankind in 1969, average Americans were probably much more inconvenienced by a bout with a cold than by the inability of humans to take a stroll on the surface of an object 240,000 miles from earth.

Similarly, in 1997, one is much more likely to hear neighbors talking over the back fence about the financial and caregiving burdens presented by aging parents than about their longing to recreate themselves, family members, household pets, or livestock in a petri dish. This is not to disparage science and the wonders it has produced. The very existence of Dolly the sheep sends my imagination into orbit. And therein lies the difference between solving the problems of daily life and boldly going where no man or woman has gone before. The latter captures our imagination, excites us with possibilities, offers hope that we can, after all, control our destiny and fulfill our dreams.

Providing for an aging nation's long term care needs, on the other hand, is something most people want to spend as little time as possible contemplating. This is not the stuff indulgent daydreams are made of. It is the stuff real life is made of, and we must begin to find real answers. If the demographers are right, the number of Americans aged 85 and older could reach 31 million by the year 2050, from just 3.1 million in 1994. We have simply run out of time for handwringing about how best to prepare for this country's current and future long term care needs.

Solving our long-term care financing crisis may not promise the immediate thrill and delight that some milestone achievements do. What it does promise, however, is improved economic security and quality of life for families, communities, and the nation—a prospect that should give us all goosebumps.

Reprinted with permission of the American Health Care Association's *Provider Magazine* (April 1997, v. 23(4):6). Copyright American Health Care Association. Edited from the original.

THE MACPHERSON TRIANGULATION TECHNIQUE

Leo A. Gordon, MD, FACS

Medical diagnosis is no longer the challenge for today's experienced physician. The real challenge is to figure out how to gain managed care approval for the studies necessary to reach a diagnosis. Physicians know how to diagnose. We know common patterns of disease, and by way of such knowledge and deductive reasoning we can come to the diagnosis. But getting there—which used to be half the fun—has now been impeded by the concept of outside approval. The creative energies, intelligence, and excitement of the diagnostic pursuit have now been channelled into the health plan approval process.

In an effort to work toward recapturing fun in medicine, let us look at today's typical scenario, and see how we might change it. When the doctor hears the patient's complaint, certain hypotheses and tests come to mind. The doctor may also know from clinical experience that the necessary investigation can best be done "outside the plan." Clinical experience is a powerful teacher in the grand scheme of medical education. But it is not a cost variable that lends itself to financial analysis. Therefore, it plays no role in the current health care equation. To get to that equation with work outside the preapproved list, the physician must seek approval.

Who does the approval? None of the plan administrators or top-level people are staffing the voice mail. They are too busy with soundproofing their offices to deaden the noise of compounding interest as it turns over from their stock options. The approvers are lower down on the administrative food chain. They live by various documents, flowsheets, and "practice plans" that can grant or deny approval for the test or for the referral.

Now for the secret of dealing with these powerful bureaucrats. As a service to my colleagues, I have formulated a method to achieve proper referral to institutions or individuals who are more expert at a particular test, yet whose approval for that test will surely be denied by the health care plan.

This method is not dishonest, illegal, or unethical. It does, as my departed father would say, merely "bend the truth a bit." Besides, we all recall the aphorism of Hippocrates: ". . . if approval is denied, yet the practitioner believes that the patient may be better served, the physician has a duty and obligation to finagle and get the proper referral."

To obtain approval, one simply uses the MacPherson Triangulation Technique. For example, a physician wants to refer a patient to a particular facility or to a particular physician, but that facility or physician is not in the plan. The physician submits the form for approval, and the approval is denied. The physician calls the responsible person, usually designated the "referral coordinator," using the following script:

"Hello, this is Dr. Gordon (the physician should use his/her own name). I wanted to refer Mrs. Jones to the Better Memorial Hospital for a needle-localized breast biopsy, and the referral was denied. The referral says she has to go to Lesser General."

"Yes, Dr. Gordon. Better Memorial is not on our referral list. That's why your request was denied."

"But the Better Memorial Hospital offers something that, in the long run, will be cheaper for your plan." (The magic word has been used, the mother lode of referral approval has instantly been tapped.)

"What is that?"

"That is the MacPherson Triangulation Technique."

"The what?"

"The MacPherson Triangulation Technique. It is a new technique that is faster, cheaper, and better for the patient. Did I mention that it was cheaper? Or the cheapest? Yes, cheaper, and cheaper for the plan, allowing a lower global fee, less hospital

---

Reprinted with permission of the author and Bulletin of the American College of Surgeons, © 1998; 83(2):35–37. Edited from the original.

usage, and less involvement with the physicians and, therefore, cheaper physician charges. Did I mention that it was less expensive or cheaper? It's low-cost, very economical, and a bargain. Did I say it was cheaper? Yes, they triangulate the patient, rather than relying on a more costly diagonal approach. I'm surprised you people haven't heard of it."

"Did you say the MacPherson Triangulation Technique was cheaper?"

"Oh, definitely, it's branching out into all kinds of tests and procedures. Many doctors are using it."

"Please hold." (Begin Kenny G music.)

We are now at a critical juncture of the approval process, where the protocol is being reviewed at the other end of the line. It is quite likely, however, that having used the word "cheap" six or seven times, the referral will be approved no matter what the protocol states. If the referral coordinator contacts a physician/manager, that physician will also approve the referral, since it is likely that he or she is no longer in practice, or if he is, it will be in a specialty unrelated to the patient's problem.

"OK, Dr. Gordon, we've approved the patient for Better Memorial Hospital based on the MacPherson Technique."

"Thank you. Please fax over the approval."

Several minutes later, the Holy Grail of managed care arrives—an out-of-plan referral approval. This document is, in busy established medical offices, undergoing the transition to managed care, akin to a Gutenberg Bible coming out of the fax machine.

Please note, dear colleagues, that the MacPherson Triangulation Technique is universal in its application. Let's say there is a needed special pathologist, radiation therapist, urologist, or even, dare I say, a surgeon who is "out of the plan." All one has to do to get the patient to that particular physician is to tell the referral coordinator that the physician uses the MacPherson Triangulation Technique. You can tailor your own scripts. For example:

"Oh, yes, Dr. Outofplan uses the MacPherson Technique for prostatectomies. The procedure is shorter, and so is the hospital stay. Did I mention that the technique is cheaper? You see he triangulates the trigone...."

Or, again:

"Oh, yes, Dr. Miles the neurologist triangulates the patient in his office using the MacPherson Technique. It cuts down on the time for exam and interview and, ultimately, on the need for hospitalization. He can see four patients using the technique in the time he used to take to see one patient. Did I mention that using the MacPherson Technique is cheaper and less expensive?"

And finally:

"Of course the patient should see Dr. Heaton for the aneurysm. Dr. Heaton triangulates the aneurysm using the MacPherson Technique before operating on it. Did I say that aneurysmectomy with Dr. Heaton was cheaper for the plan?"

And so on and so on.

Implementing the MacPherson Triangulation Technique for out-of-plan referral takes some practice. One must speak the words in a serious manner. Seminars are being held throughout our great nation on the use of this technique for better patient care. (I feel the need to break out into a focus group right now!)

To get a patient into a particular facility—one with which you have had a good experience—just use the MacPherson Triangulation Technique.

By the way, I am always available for consultation. If I am not on the roster or am "out of plan," just tell the referral coordinator that "Dr. Gordon triangulates the gallbladder, which allows him to...."

A CLINIC FOR EVERYONE

Robert M. Goldwyn, MD

"Of course, it will work," proclaimed C. Bottom Lygne, executive director of The Hospital, to I. M. Duterful, his associate director. "The country is moving in the direction of splintering, and I intend to help it along. Gone are the days of the old-time clinics—what I call the generic clinics—you remember, the Gastrointestinal Clinic, the Urological Clinic—to get patients, we have to have specific clinics."

"Maybe you're right," intoned Duterful, whose six-figure income depended on telling his boss that he was always right. "I admit that I was skeptical when you broke down the GI Clinic into 22 subclinics: The GI Clinic for Divorced Men, the one for Left Handers, and the one for Retired Postal Clerks between the ages of 73 and 79."

"I sensed a tidal wave of phony consumerism was coming and I rode it in," bragged CEO Lygne, leaning back in a chair larger than anything in Buckingham Palace. "You see, Duterful, this country is falsely called the United States. No longer is the motto *E Pluribus Unum*, 'Out of Many One'—it really should be 'Out of One, Many.' We have thousands, maybe millions of groups of people, each demanding their rights. Responsibilities went out with the end of Prohibition, as far as I can see. Women want their own medical care by women. Men, so far, are bewildered, but I predict soon they will want a 'Men's Health Center Run of Men, by Men, and for Men.' And, Duterful, you and I and this hospital will be in the forefront. Think of it. We will have clinics for those of every background: Polish, Armenian, Icelandic, Samoan. We already have a Native American Clinic. We will have clinics for those of every skin hue. We will match doctors and nurses with patients by spectrophotometry. We might even get into religion and philosophy—you know, a subclinic for every belief, perhaps one even for agnostics and atheists. There is no limit to this except what the human mind can devise. I have turned this challenge over to our Computer Department so that they can give us all possible permutations."

"Aren't you becoming a bit extreme?" added Duterful, an unusually brave statement from him, but now he was concerned that if Bottom Lygne became too grandiose, the Board of Trustees might terminate him, and he also would lose his job.

"In this country," replied Bottom Lygne, with a measured voice and a firm look, "you can never go far enough in recognizing minute entities. The melting pot concept was totally wrong from the beginning. Each ingredient in the so-called pot has always remained distinct."

"Wouldn't we have to increase the number of personnel considerably to provide all these options for patients?"

"To some degree, yes, but people can play double or multiple roles. It is possible, for example, to find a person of Bulgarian descent who is an agnostic as well as left-handed. That individual can serve in three clinics. It is all a matter of planning, my dear Duterful. I used to think that progress in medicine depended on research and discoveries; it is really a matter of marketing. Yes, from time to time an advance comes along, but disease and death always win. That is why health care providers will always be needed. Maybe we won't be called that in the future, but someone has to be there to bring doctors and patients together. Also, keep in mind that people don't have to be ill to be patients. With the emphasis now on prevention, everyone is a patient. We will get even the healthiest in this country to lie awake nights fearing a mortal disease by the morning."

"Bottom Lygne, you are a genius," Duterful says, meaning it.

"No, just an incorrigible realist," his boss replies with cultivated modesty.

Reprinted with permission from Plastic and Reconstructive Surgery, © 1994; 94(5):699.

HAL REVISITED

Mary Grayson

The movie *2001: A Space Odyssey* gave many of us our first glimpse at what a computerized future might look like. We sat mesmerized by the beautiful classical music, coordinated with the stunning visions of outer space, and were lulled into contentment by the soothing, reassuring voice of Hal, the "flawless" HAL Series 9000 supercomputer that runs and monitors all of the spaceship's higher and lower functions. Hal is also good at chess.

As I'm sure you recall, the intrepid space voyagers are called to the moon because a mysterious object has been found buried in a lunar crater. This is a very big deal because none of the space-savvy scientists know what the object is. However, they are certain it predates the human race. Today, such an event would be enough to drive all of mankind into a frenzy, launch several new tabloid newspapers overnight, and keep Mulder and Scully in a state of high anxiety and sleeplessness for the rest of their television lives.

Predictably, the spacemen can't leave well enough alone. They just have to know what the object is, so they set to work with their little lunar shovels and dig it up. Shortly after being unearthed, the monolith begins shrieking, sending signals to Jupiter, and causing all sorts of mysterious trouble. (Next time listen to the folks at the electric company: Call before you dig!)

Most people, including myself, left the theater puzzled by what the monolith was or what it symbolized. Years later while listening to late-night talk radio, I realized what the monolith stood for: national health insurance. It was deliberately buried on the moon by opponents in hopes that no one would ever uncover it again and be attracted to its siren song. (Now, admit it. Doesn't that make perfect sense? Why, with a little research, I bet we could prove that the all-purpose prophet Nostradamus actually predicted this.)

Of course, the real star of *2001* is Hal. He is considered a villain, but let's be fair. Hal's downfall is his human tendencies, not his technology. He does an excellent job of keeping everything running smoothly until he goes insane. The spacemen on the voyage to Jupiter don't really have much to do except jog and write notations in their daily total quality management time logs, such as "Didn't do much today—again," "Nada," and "Ditto."

Granted, Hal has that little bad spell there when he makes a few mistakes, tries to sabotage the entire mission, gives the spacemen inaccurate information, locks them out of their own ship, flings one into the abyss, murders three others in their sleep, and eventually kills all the spacemen except one. But hey, we've all worked with human beings like that. At least Hal is polite.

Before the dawn of the actual computer age, Hal represented what many of us thought computers would do for us—that is to say, everything. We would be only minimally involved, and everything would run smoothly. Our expectations were a tad unrealistic. Since then, we've all occasionally harbored murderous thoughts about our info systems, and I suspect some companies returned the favor.

Computer technology is an industry developing at a dazzling speed, but it's still a developing industry. Look how long it took the auto industry—and how loudly consumers had to yell—before GM, Ford, and Chrysler stopped adding fins and made a reliable car. Many a sun set behind the mountain.

But lo! 2001 is at hand, and vendors and health care execs are ready to embark on a new odyssey of shared risk. Maybe this time everyone will get there alive—and well.

Reprinted from *Hospitals & Health Networks*, Vol. 72, No. 4, by permission, February 20, 1998. Copyright 1998, by Health Forum, Inc.

WHAT IT REALLY MEANS

Maybe it's just a function of getting older, but nothing seems straightforward anymore. We've manufactured a whole new vocabulary to cover all of life's nasty events, so that now even the worst scenario seems benign. Restructuring just sounds so much better than saying that half of the employees won't be here a year from now. Being downsized has a nice ring to it, like finally managing to shed those last pesky ten pounds, rather than being fired. So, the next time the scuttlebutt is that your organization will be merged, reorganized, or affiliated, hold onto your hats, it's going to be a bumpy ride.

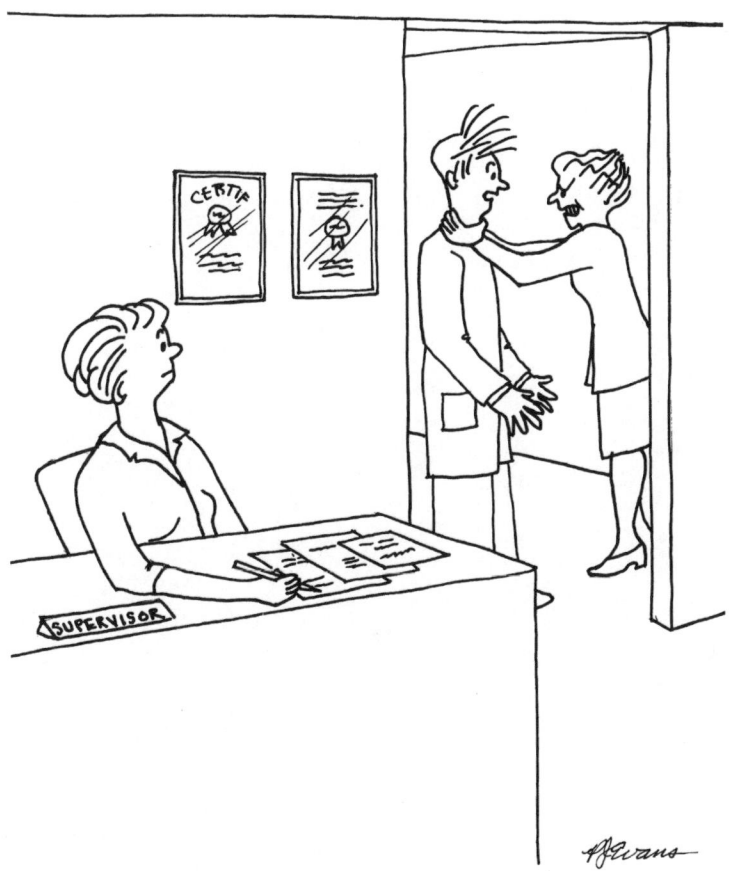

"Time to write another job ad for this cooperative, team-oriented, and motivating environment."

CAN WE TALK?

Elizabeth A. J. Hasegawa, PharmD

The electronic information age is here, and its impact on society is magnificent, encroaching, and undeniable. Manipulating information and passing it simultaneously to more individuals than ever before will continue to be hailed as great progress and will change how we think about many things. Our definitions of the learning process and of librarians, for example, are evolving rapidly. Even the definition of communication has been altered to accommodate our new abilities to move words, pictures, and sounds. Today, dictionaries define communication first as imparting information. Other terms follow, however, such as "rapport," "conversing," and "exchange." Accepting the latter terms means accepting that communication does not exist without replies that describe the understanding of all parties.

Frequently, all we need is the simple act of informing, but for the more important aspects of our profession and our lives, we should hold communication to be a discourse that proceeds logically from a point of mystery to a point of clarity. Mistaking information delivery for complete communication could produce effects opposite those for which much of our new technology is promoted: improving our understanding of others and enabling us to apply our understanding in productive ways. Indeed, there are signs that, rather than bringing people closer via better understanding, our reliance on the computer is separating us and stunting our abilities to engage each other in meaningful conversation.

The institution where I work has offered a seminar called "How To Deal with Difficult People." The mission of a department includes educating its staff about communication because we do not get the practice we need in daily life. The profession of "facilitator" has recently emerged, complete with an international society to represent it. A facilitator, who is paid $1500 to $4500 a day, essentially behaves as the "grownup," trying to get groups of dissenting persons to communicate.

Using e-mail—avoiding conversation because it is easier to remain seated and type a message—is only the most egregious example of how opportunities to practice communication skills are wasted. It is common for e-mail to be received from 10 feet away. Proponents say it saves time, but I question whether the majority of e-mail has resulted in free time in which something else was actually produced. Indeed, it is not inconceivable that much time is consumed explaining e-mail messages to skeptical and indignant recipients. All parties in such episodes would have benefited personally and professionally from spoken conversation.

Conversation does not always require one-on-one meetings to be useful; the old-fashioned staff meeting should provide an excellent venue for explaining, listening, and responding. The staff meetings I remember involved lots of talking, listening, comparing notes, and even some table banging. It was communication that traveled back and forth, and understanding (or lack of it) could be judged immediately. When the meeting was over, there might not have been agreement, but the topic was digested and remembered. It was not always easy or even pleasant, but it was excellent practice. Lessons learned face-to-face apply widely in life, whereas sending an e-mail teaches absolutely nothing about how to be understood (although the reactions of some recipients may be very educational).

Another illustration of our failure to practice communicating is provided by the ubiquitous CD-ROM. One, entitled Dr. Scheuler's Home Medical Advisor Pro ($100), provides possible diagnoses and advice after a person enters his or her symptoms. It is information en masse in the privacy of home, away from white coats, the office, people, the world. But is it communication? Is it education? Is so much information in isolation conducive to good

Reprinted with permission from American Journal of Health-System Pharmacy, © 1997; 54(5):584–585. Edited from the original.

health? A reviewer wrote of this particular CD-ROM: "It understands that patients have symptoms, not systems." It does? That is impressive for a piece of vinyl. It is even more impressive if such an object is filling a vacuum created by health professionals' inability or unwillingness to converse and to ensure understanding. This is not an example of technology enhancing or taking over a person's job. It's a case of loads of information being mistaken for communication. A CD-ROM makes an elegant package for information, but it does not judge how the information has been understood or how it will or will not be applied to the user's situation. In other words, it does not communicate. Do we?

Technology and computers have their place. Undoubtedly, distributing items such as meeting minutes and announcements electronically has saved time and paper and is a huge improvement over hours spent manually copying and distributing. Electronic files are not necessarily easier to find than papers in a file cabinet, but they do occupy less space. But let's use computers for tasks they do better than we: storing, displaying, and disseminating information. Let's not tolerate them as substitutes for human communication.

I have been working in hospitals for 20 years. I have never learned anything about my profession from a videotape or a CD-ROM that I did not learn better from a person. The ability to send and receive e-mail has not made me a better pharmacist, but conversing with a person has. Dashing off an e-mail message after a problematic event has not brought long-lasting satisfaction, nor has it improved patient care. However, investing the time to address differences face-to-face has accomplished both. The opportunities to practice genuine communication are becoming too precious to let e-mail take their place.

In some circles, the phrase "use it or lose it" refers to paid time off. It also applies to any skill that takes practice, including face-to-face conversation between human beings. Let's keep electronically passed information in its place and restore the vanishing art of talking with each other.

EFFECT ON HUMAN LONGEVITY OF ADDED DIETARY CHOCOLATE

Joel Kirschbaum, PhD

Introduction

The working hypothesis is that the general feeling of well-being derived from the delectable taste of chocolate would lead to a more positive outlook on life. It is well documented that happier individuals have significantly higher serum concentrations of γ-immunoglobulin. Increased quantities of immunoglobulins would, in turn, improve the ability of the immune system to interact and interfere with both invading bacteria and aberrant, abnormal cells, which would be reflected in an enhanced lifespan.

Reprinted from Nutrition, 14(11/12), 869, © 1998, with permission from Elsevier Science.

Experimental

The experimental protocol involved feeding either imitation chocolate (control group) or various quantities of 40% cocoa butterfat-content dark chocolate over a 10-y span to a statistically significant population, and following mortality. Analyses of the dark chocolate for authenticity involved daily organoleptic testing, which was the initial motivation for this study, following a previous protocol involving studying the beneficial effects of supplementing diets with lobster and champagne.

Results and Discussion

The data demonstrated that moderate daily additions of dark, 40% butterfat-content chocolate increased both average lifespans and γ-immunoglobulin concentrations compared with the control group. The maximum average lifespan extension of 4 y was achieved by the addition to the diet of 4 kg chocolate per 50 kg body weight/mo. However, higher supplemental quantities from 4 to 8 kg resulted in lesser average lifespan enhancements until no difference in average longevity was found between the 8 kg of added chocolate/mo group and the control subjects. The dose-response curve was not bell-shaped but Hershey Kiss-shaped; giving new meaning to the term "kiss of life." (Here, CPR means not cardiopulmonary resuscitation but chocolate per repast.) Above 8 kg chocolate/mo, the average lifespan decreased to below that of the control group, even ignoring the effect on the data of several experimental subjects who either tripped over or fell off the scale and crushed themselves. However, anecdotal evidence indicates that all members of the "excess" chocolate group died with smiles on their faces. The life-shortening effects of "excess" chocolate may indicate the inability of the high concentrations of chocolate-induced γ-immunoglobulin cells to squeeze past plaque-coated capillaries, and thus interact and interfere with internal invaders.

The implications of these findings are obvious. Individuals should add M & M's to their vitamin pill piles. Governments must decide to either allow chocolate purchases to be medical deductions from income taxes or (because it can be argued that chocoholics will live longer and thus collect greater total pensions) institute a surcharge on chocolate. Finally, the morbidly obese should be taxed, per extra pound, with these revenues reserved for lower income individuals to supplement food stamps with fudge stamps.

WORDS THAT DENY REALITY

Jules M. Rothstein, PhD, PT, FAPTA

Language is supposed to be a means by which sentient beings capable of cognition communicate ideas, concepts, commands, and concrete images. But lurking beneath it all lies the human penchant for avoidance, lily gilding, and self-serving prose. During an otherwise delightful meal in a Philadelphia restaurant, this became obvious to me. The pretentiously oversized menu should have set me up for what was to follow, but I was still surprised by the first item, "Thai-style Cappellini." That's one heck of a concept. "Italian-style Curry" was not on the menu, but the second item was some dish with a "young baby chicken." A young baby chicken? Were they talking about deviled eggs?

The food was great, but every item on the menu was described in breathlessly inexact prose. Was there a fear that food for thought would be so filling that customers would not order a decent meal? Whatever happened to descriptive menus that told you what you were ordering? Menus have become more pompous than Henry Kissinger and equally candid in telling you what they represent, and as a result there are lots of nice-sounding words carefully strung together to provide images that really describe nothing.

Restaurants are not alone in using words to avoid reality. As I recently bounced around in a commuter plane crossing the frighteningly high Wasatch Mountains, I made the mistake of consulting Skywest's in-flight magazine. There I learned that the plane I was in offered "An intimate cabin with many advantages of larger aircraft, the 19-passenger Metro allows every passenger to enjoy both a window and an aisle seat." In other words, the

Reprinted from Physical Therapy, © 1994; 74(7):611–613, with the permission of the APTA. Edited from the original.

circumference of the fuselage is so small there are two narrow seats separated by an aisle that bears a striking resemblance to the gutter that lies along a bowling lane.

I can see why the airline felt a need to avoid an accurate description. On the Metro, passengers get to recapitulate evolution by knuckle walking on and off because they dare not walk *Homo sapiens* style for fear of crashing their skulls into the roof of the cabin. Buy why couldn't the airline avoid the temptation to obfuscate and simply say that the small plane allowed for service that would not otherwise be financially feasible to communities in need of an air service?

My concern is that we have become accustomed to using language to avoid reality. The strategy in the restaurant and for the airline was not to describe, but rather to hide and to pander. Tell people what they want to hear, and they might see the world differently. Hot sauce being a dangerous condiment, I recently read the labels on two different brands, only to see the following strange ingredient: "edible food stabilizers." I was comforted to know they hadn't added *in*edible food stabilizers, but then I realized edibility should be the consumer's judgment. And then I really understood what they were talking about. Gone were all those nasty chemical names people hate to see, and in their place was not a description, but rather a conclusion.

This business of using words for the purpose of not communicating is as old as Adam and Eve. A careful re-reading of Genesis reveals that more than a fair share of characters tried to fool God with careful linguistic feats of derring-do (remember, for example, the purpose of asking, "Am I my brother's keeper?"). Apparently, we are in a good company when we are on the receiving end of slippery prose offered in lieu of communication.

Unfortunately, airlines, restaurants, and hot-sauce purveyors are not the only ones who know how to use words to steer us clear of understanding or to puff up communications. Think of the phrases we serve up daily in notes and verbal dalliances. Patients *deny* things when in reality they simply say they never had something. We talk of *symptomatology* when "symptoms" would do, and of course we incorrectly use the word *parameter* whenever possible, even though more suitable words abound. There are *parameters* for electrical stimulation because it is too mundane to talk about *machine settings*, and we study parameters of gait because if we talked about *variables*, our fancy equipment might seem less fancy.

Actually, my favorite silly usage occurs when we talk about *presenting* with things. I just cannot shake the image of the credit roll before those old movie spectaculars when giant letters proclaimed that some producer was presenting something. Did Mrs. Schwartz really present with a hip fracture à la a Las Vegas chorus line, or did she just have a hip fracture?

Enough with the complaining and whining on my part—as Genesis attests, even more powerful beings than journal editors have had little effect on getting others to behave. So what can we do to stop the fanciful juxtaposition of usage and meaning? Perhaps we need to turn elsewhere and accept that not only will peace begin with each of us, but so will the proper use of language.

I am tempted to call for a modern version of the Spanish Inquisition featuring black-robed inquisitors holding each of us accountable for the words we use. But such a call goes against my nature and, more importantly, use of the metaphor alone might make me vulnerable to one of their early purges. Let me instead just paraphrase a recent plea and ask, "Can't we just communicate? Can't we all just try to communicate with each other?"

TIPS FOR INTERPRETING "SCIENCE-SPEAK"

"IT HAS LONG BEEN KNOWN"
... I didn't look up the original reference.

"A DISTINCT TREND IS EVIDENT"
... These data are practically meaningless.

"WHILE IT HAS NOT BEEN POSSIBLE TO PROVIDE DEFINITE ANSWERS TO THESE QUESTIONS"
... An unsuccessful experiment, but I still hope to get it published.

"THREE OF THE SAMPLES WERE CHOSEN FOR DETAILED STUDY"
... The results of the others did not make any sense.

"TYPICAL RESULTS ARE SHOWN"
... This is the prettiest graph.

"THESE RESULTS WILL BE IN A SUBSEQUENT REPORT"
... I might get around to this sometime, if pushed/funded.

"THE MOST RELIABLE RESULTS ARE OBTAINED BY JONES"
... He was my graduate student; his grade depended on this.

"IN MY EXPERIENCE"
... Once.

"IN CASE AFTER CASE"
... Twice.

"IN A SERIES OF CASES"
... Thrice.

"IT IS BELIEVED THAT"
... I think.

"IT IS GENERALLY BELIEVED THAT"
... A couple of other guys think so too.

"CORRECT WITHIN AN ORDER OF MAGNITUDE"
... Wrong.

"ACCORDING TO STATISTICAL ANALYSIS"
... Rumor has it.

"A STATISTICALLY ORIENTED PROJECTION OF THE SIGNIFICANCE OF THESE FINDINGS"
... A wild guess.

"A CAREFUL ANALYSIS OF OBTAINABLE DATA"
... Three pages of notes were obliterated when I knocked over a glass of beer.

"IT IS CLEAR THAT MUCH ADDITIONAL WORK WILL BE REQUIRED BEFORE A COMPLETE UNDERSTANDING OF THIS PHENOMENON OCCURS"
... I don't understand it.

"AFTER ADDITIONAL STUDY BY MY COLLEAGUES"
... They don't understand it either.

"THANKS ARE DUE TO JOE BLOTZ FOR ASSISTANCE WITH THE EXPERIMENT AND TO ANDREA SCHAEFFER FOR VALUABLE DISCUSSIONS"
... Mr. Blotz did the work and Ms. Schaeffer explained to me what it meant.

"A HIGHLY SIGNIFICANT AREA FOR EXPLORATORY STUDY"
... A totally useless topic selected by my committee.

Downloaded from the Internet and reprinted with permission from Research Nurse, © 1996; 2(6):18.

BITS, BYTES, AND MIDDLE AGE

Victor Ince, ART

A widely held theory states that "Laboratories require more young people to adapt to computerized technology." It is irrefutable that the newly graduated medical technologist is required to perform effectively in a laboratory where most equipment is controlled by microchip technology.

The problem is not with this theory, but rather with the presumptions stemming from interpolation of the theory.

The middle aged department head, chief technologist, or laboratory manager is fearful of his or her ability to reach retirement age with a job intact.

This, of course, is not a theory, rather the widely held hypothesis of the previously mentioned bright eyed new graduates. Considering that the average fifty-year-old technologist was trained in the dark age of burette chemistry, there appears to be ample evidence to support the thesis.

Most of the equipment we used then is not quite old enough to be considered for museum display, but it is just so much junk in today's laboratory store room.

The middle-aged staff, trained in such an archaic environment, can hardly be expected to grasp the intricacies of microchip technology.

The first step toward restoring reality is to look at what has happened to the new graduate during training, and to the older technologist during the last twenty-five (plus) years in the clinical laboratory.

Today's academic student receives an exposure to computers in most high schools. After graduation comes a more rapid immersion into the manipulation of statistical data by computers. The majority of the programs used are menu driven. Programming is not a significant part of medical technology training.

These machines have taken over the time-consuming and exacting tasks of pipetting, sample selection, report transcription, and many more. They trouble shoot, and they type reports; they check our spelling and can even fix our grammar.

Today's graduate spends more and more time placing small cups of serum on the analyzer and carrying printed reports to the charge technologist for checking. Each new labor intensive test procedure which breaks the monotony seems to be rapidly replaced with an automated computer-controlled system "to eliminate the chance of error."

The new graduate is also full of the joys of youth. Skiing, hiking, sailing, and traveling replace, augment, or complement The Hunt. In the first few years of work the most important part of the day is going home to play.

The laboratory elders, on the other hand, have learned to perform all tasks manually. They have learned to write a report correctly the first time, or face the wrath of a secretary who had no qualms stating her resentment about having to retype anything.

Every small step in automation was a struggle, and every ill-conceived technological nightmare was an education never anticipated in college. Every technologist's problems are different although they all share a common thread.

A new graduate presenting a simple straightforward solution to a perennial laboratory problem is often overwhelmed by the number of problems which roll off the tongue of the older technologists, almost without a moment's reflection.

There is certainly a great deal of truth in one adage, "Old age and treachery can always overcome youth and skill!" Another adage is less appropriate: "You can't teach an old dog new tricks!"

Despite, or perhaps because of, the younger technologist's exposure to computers, there seems to be very little interest in the workings of these, now essential, devices. The input of data and the

---

Reprinted from Canadian Journal of Medical Technology, © 1990; 52(3):143–144, with permission of the author. Edited from the original.

distribution of completed reports seem to satisfy. There is, of course, an appreciation of the troubleshooting aspects of instrumentation incorporating this feature.

After considerable non-scientific, random research coupled with first-hand observation, the writer has observed an interesting phenomenon. It is not the young who are immersed in computers, rather it is the middle-aged and older technologists.

The result of this phenomena is that the younger technologists are very dependent on the older technologists when any computer problem arises. From the generation of new spread sheets for unit calculation to the design of a new requisition, there is ready acceptance that the person best able to perform the task received their education years before the man in the street even heard the word computer.

Perhaps the question should be asked, "Does the middle-aged staff accept the lack of initiative of young technologists?"

To this question the answer is undoubtedly YES. Those aging middle-aged technologists recognize that education is not complete with the granting of an RT. The newly graduated medical technologist has just achieved a very basic understanding of medical technology.

The first day on the job marks the beginning of a new phase of higher education which will go on for the rest of each individual's life. After 30 years of the world of work the middle-aged technologists appreciate how far the new graduate has to go and will be content to let them learn at their own speed.

There is another factor which influences the older technologist's decision not to rush the new graduate. We have found this new tool, the computer! We are comfortable in our jobs and we are ready to take on a new challenge.

For now the laboratory elders do not have to fear the skills of the more junior staff. Neither one is standing still. As the elders teach, both groups learn. The rapidly expanding body of knowledge assures the continuing interest and attention of both old and young.

MEDIA LAMENT

Karen H. Morin, DSN, RN

I have seen too many well-known speakers present their visuals in a poor, distracting, or unprofessional manner. The following poem was written as a friendly, funny reminder to the reader to take care as they prepare and use visual aids.

Busy slides, oh no!
How could this be so?

Blank screen,
Unsightly scene,
Again and again.
Oh, such pain!

Using transparencies
Without sensitivities
For one's eyesight!
Oh, what a fright!

Illustrious speakers,
Established speakers,
Why such bleepers?

Is it that
They just don't know
How to show
Information to the best?
Or is the presenter in distress?

Ah, perhaps the problem is
Just not time
To do the job
Just fine!

Reprinted with permission from Journal of Continuing Education in Nursing, © 1998; 28(2):96.

ON THE OTHER SIDE OF THE RESEARCH LOOKING GLASS

Mark Radcliffe

On the other side of the research looking glass, Mark Radcliffe finds hedgehogs crossing the road wearing little fluorescent jackets and wonders what we are to do with this knowledge.

How do you measure the worth of a piece of research? Is it valued according to its methodological rigour; the career or educational advances it affords its author; or how meaningful it might be in the world? Let's think about the hedgehogs.

A long-term study in the north of England into hedgehog morbidity and road craft is, for me, something of a model of how the gathering of facts through the application of science makes the world a more understandable place.

Apparently researchers, admirably concerned for the well-being of hedgehogs, began to investigate why so many of them got squashed by passing cars. They quickly discovered, using something like a randomised-controlled trial that more hedgehogs got squashed on the bends than on the straights. They extended their research and finally concluded that "more hedgehogs get squashed on the bends because the hedgehogs can't see the cars coming and the cars can't see the hedgehogs."

A closer look at the research, its method, its significance and its relevance is, I understand, the thing to do.

Half the hedgehogs were given little fluorescent jackets and the other half were not given a damn thing. This caused problems, obviously. A fight broke out between a couple of the more headstrong hedgehogs, because Harry split some milk over Henry's jacket. Later those hedgehogs who had not been allocated a jacket threatened to walk out on the whole shebang until the researchers offered them all nice hats.

Of course this caused problems for the researchers: how could they be sure that the hedgehog hats would not interfere with the research? The hedgehogs claimed that they often wore hats so "what's the big deal" but, as the researchers rightly pointed out, they would say that wouldn't they. A compromise was reached. The hedgehogs would keep the hats, but would take them off while crossing the road.

Ethical questions were raised. Who can say which hedgehog deserved the fluorescent jacket? The researchers may have known they were condemning the hat-wearing hedgehogs to certain death. Should they say anything? One researcher remarked: "We'd go out for a drink after work and some of the prickly fellas would tell us of their little hedgehog dreams and we'd know, if they had a hat on, that they were probably not going to pull through. But in the interests of science we'd keep quiet."

The hedgehogs of course had their own ideas: "More straight roads, fewer cars. Maybe little helmets for us... We miss the Romans. You knew where you were with the Romans. Smashing roads, nice togas and pizza."

There were rumours that some time during the research some of the hedgehogs disappeared in the night, wary of the outcome of the upcoming trial. Consequently the whole project ran the risk of having no statistical significance. It has been claimed that the researchers hired some unsuspecting stoats and glued lots of combs to their backs. The problem was that stoats run faster than hedgehogs so they only hired old stoats, or stoats who limped. The researchers deny this charge most vigorously.

A lot of innocent hedgehogs died that day, as did one or two stoats and for what? What are we going to do with this knowledge? The researchers had one

Reproduced by kind permission of Nursing Times where this article first appeared, June 17, 1998; 94(24):26. Edited from the original.

of two ways to go. Either recommending investment in little hedgehog bridges or at least some appropriate traffic control system. Or they could concentrate on educating the prickly little fellas. There are problems with both of these. On the one hand, who is going to pay for little hedgehog bridges? You could have some kind of toll system I suppose and eventually the bridge will pay for itself, but who is going to put up the money in the first place and how many hedgehogs carry cash these days? In terms of education, the main problem is how many teachers speak hedgehog? And anyway hedgehogs are notoriously poor students. How many hedgehogs do you know with A levels?

THE BEEPER, AND ITS USE IN MATING DISPLAYS

Bruce Carlson

Recent research indicates that, contrary to previous theories, what separates man from animal is not the ability to use fire, or language, or even the desire to trim his own nose hairs.

It is the ability to leave messages.

Only humans can inform other humans that they are going to stop and pick up dinner on the way home from work, and do it (leave the message) almost completely without spraying urine anywhere. Indeed, once early humans had developed language, there is some evidence the first words actually spoken were "Hi! You've reached Jim—and Barbara—Slothpoker, but we're not home right now..."

And as human brains evolved into larger and larger organs, messaging abilities increased along with them. Indeed, according to ABC News, today, modern man gets an average of 169 messages a day.

The culmination of all this has been the pager, a small device worn mainly on the belt, which has completely eliminated the need to sniff fire hydrants for data, although it has created other distinctive displays. People lurch suddenly, and for no apparent reason plunge their hands into their pants. Naturalists report countless observations of individuals in face to face conversation, one party saying, "I see by the smoke pouring from your head that your hair is on fire," and the other, because her beeper is going off, responding only with a glassy expression, and vague hand movements towards her waist.

Pagers are now displayed prominently, indicating status and reproductive availability, not unlike personalized license plates. You can always tell who the alpha beeper is in a group of corporate executives, as he or she always gets the most frequent—and longest—messages, and is always able to drive the young bucks away from any available public phones.

Survival-wise, this works better for the executives, as they no longer have to risk physical injury by butting heads or inflating throat sacks in dominance duels over corner offices.

If you don't believe me about this, just look at what happened the day the pagers died.

This happened last May, when the Galaxy IV, a satellite that appears to have been named after a '71 Ford, had a massive computer failure while floating some 22,500 miles over Kansas. Everyone's beeper screen lit up with "IMPORTANT SERVICE MESSAGE: DUE TO TECHNICAL DIFFICULTIES AHHHHH! HELP ME! SWEET JESUS, HELP ME!"

The author of this paper was at an airport when it happened, and can report firsthand remarkable similarities to the movies *Deep Impact* and *Armageddon*, just with less attractive rioters. People were

Reprinted with permission from Journal of Irreproducible Results, © 1998; 43(5/6):51–52. Edited from the original.

observed poking, shaking, and cursing, both their pagers and each other. There were howls of rage into cellular phones and incoherent sobbing in the arms of traveling companions, all at a level unseen since the last big Beanie Babies sale.

Prior to this incident we knew that in humans, the individual with the most messages was the most dominant; that Beepers evolved past their simple message function to become more like moose antlers, which are displayed prominently during mating season. We just hadn't realized how big and moss-covered the human racks had become.

As a determinant of breeding desirability, beepers have proven themselves superior to other display methods. They can be shown on the person anywhere, indoors or out, like a peacock's tail feathers. While many scientists were watching cell phones, believing them to be the markers of dominance in bureaucratic packs, pagers were appearing on more and more individuals, becoming the subject of increasingly frequent preening and grooming displays. Until now they're a more accurate dominance indicator than secretary size.

Observations, of course, continue, in hopes of spotting the early appearance of the next display mechanism. (Palm Pilots have been suggested, for instance.) But final measurements of the beepers' importance remain to be taken sometime next February, when data will be gathered on what the crash last May did to breeding statistics.

SLEEP RESEARCH UPDATE

Yuska-Marie Paskevitch

RESEARCH GROUP 1
   KD is sleeping with RM.
   RM is sleeping with PI.
   PI is sleeping with RK.
   RK is sleeping with WB.
   WB is sleeping with GG.
   GG is sleeping with FP.
   FP is sleeping with KD.

RESEARCH GROUP 3
   TFD reports a string of disappointing results. She is seeking an improved research protocol.

RESEARCH GROUP 4
   DS is breaking in a new graduate student.

RESEARCH GROUP 7
   FL has been experimenting with hair dyes.

RESEARCH GROUP 7
   KD lost his research grant, and is not sleeping with anyone.

Reprinted with permission from various issues of Annals of Improbable Research.

DON'T PUT YOUR FOOTNOTES IN YOUR MOUTH[1]

David[2] Wolman, PA-C[3]

No one seems to know how the concept of footnotes was inflicted on the unsuspecting scholar.[4] Rumor has it that footnotes were discovered by podiatrists.[5] However, pressure was brought to bear by the union of podiatrists, which is an affiliate of the Teamsters. The rumor was quelled.[6] Others thought osteopaths, early ancestors of humanoids, were responsible for the superscript digits, but this was disproved by Mary Leaky when she found an older bone in Duluth.[7] The Centers for Disease Control, on the other hand, or foot, as the case may be, hypothesizes that footnotes are viruses that were unleashed by illegal bulldozing in Newark, New Jersey, in 1955, when the city was being considered as a nuclear test sight but was already too radioactive.[8]

Alfred North Whitehead added to the general confusion by describing the history of philosophy as "simply a series of footnotes to Plato."[9] However, Plato did not use footnotes.[10] He just wrote down whatever was on his mind and he didn't even have a laptop. In fact, he stole from Socrates quite liberally, a man who walked around in bare feet and couldn't afford sandals or Dr. Scholl's footnotes. As a final insult, he was given hemlock for allegedly plagiarizing the youth.[11] Video of this was shown recently on *Real Stories of the Highway Patrol*.

Homer, too, did not use a single footnote in the entire *Iliad*,[12] despite some pretty unsubstantiated accusations about Troy, New York.

When To and When Not To

Irrespective of their historic genealogy, when do you use footnotes and when do you not? In simple terms, if there are turkey prints in the snow then there must be turkeys somewhere.[13] What that has to do with footnotes is questionable, but the statement was footnoted properly, which gives it a certain air of authority and importance whether or not it is irrelevant.

Obviously, if you are writing a poem, you do not need to use footnotes.[14] PAs do not, in the course of their daily work, have to write many poems, unless you consider a SOAP note a kind of poem. For example, here is an entry from a major medical center:
  Vital signs are okay
  Head ear eyes nose and throat are clear
  Respiratory effort blasé
  Abdomen suggestive of too much beer
  Neuro exam with no focal signs
  Extremities edematous and smelly
  Skin remarkable for lots of lines
  Assessment: too much belly

In scientific writing, footnotes are required and there are strict punishments for not using them, including a form of professional pillory, and, in some cases, a fate worse then death—misplacing your CME logging form.[15] Even after you have added every footnote you can think of, however, your editor will no doubt ask for more footnotes. That is because editors are paid by the footnote.[16]

Peer reviewers, by the way, get into the act by sending incomprehensible E-mail to you from unknown cyberspace stations asking for footnotes for your footnotes. Have you ever met a peer reviewer? I agree with Groucho Marx when he said that anyone who would peer review him was not someone he would want for a peer. I lost my taste for peers after members of KISS were made peers of the realm, though what realm was not specified.

Issues of Infringement

Some people have asked the question: if you merely copy an entire article but footnote every sentence, does that make that article your original work, as long as you use a different title, or does this fall into

Used with permission from Physician Assistant, © 1997; 21(7):80,82, Springhouse Corporation/www.springnet.com

the realm of a "reprint," which requires a little annoying "c" for copyright rather than a little annoying number for footnote? Thus, there seems to be some blurring of the lines between bootlegging, pirating, and referencing, all of which result from the illegal fermentation of too many ideas.[17] There is just too much information out there, too many smart people and too many footnotes. Someone should do something about it.

The state of all this informational referenced entropy is summarized by the expression "to err is human, but to be human is to err." At least, John Milton thought that.[18] But he forgot to use footnotes, so paradise was lost. The Bible, too, has no authorial footnotes but everyone else has gotten into the act by adding their own. And Webster's dictionary, yes Webster's, not a single footnote! Where do they get off dictating the very meaning of the words we use to construct footnotes WITH NO FOOTNOTES? And *Gray's Anatomy*? No footnotes. How do we know the thigh bone *is* connected to the hip bone?

The Long Trail

Another problem is how to footnote something that is footnoted in another article. Ideally, one should have the original source to make sure it has been ripped off appropriately.[19] A recent experiment demonstrated that 80% of footnotes misrepresent the views of the person footnoted, were in many cases gross distortions or manipulated syntax, and caused great agony for the original author, who had stolen most of his or her material or manufactured footnotes or just used rumors they had overheard in the locker room.

There is also the issue of the lag time between the completion of a manuscript and the publication of the same.[20] Recently, I was sent a galley of a manuscript to proof that I had no recollection of writing due to the fact that my article had sat on the slush pile for years because I was bumped by twelve osteoporosis articles. Has anyone actually seen osteoporosis? No hard feelings, pardon the pun, but meanwhile the information in my absolutely essential treatise entitled *Insect Life in Ear Canals* was all moldy and the footnotes were from out-of-print journals. When I searched for updated footnotes, I realized that the article no longer matched the footnotes, the cart was pulling the horse, as it were, so I had to begin all over again. That was when I began to detest those impertinent little numbers. At night, my dreams began to have footnotes and I often awoke in the morning muttering "Ibid." in my sleep. My wife said I sounded like a studious frog.

Where does one draw the line between common knowledge and footnoteability? What is common knowledge anyway? If I were to say, for example, that the sun rises in the East and sets in the West, would I need a footnote? Some would say that on Saturn my statement would be false and therefore I should reference a more competent source than myself.[21] Then there is personal opinion, which has been going out of style for years.[22] Medical articles steer away from personal opinion like the plague, limiting themselves to brief redundant introductions followed by dry, consecutive, scientific, autistic-sounding serial incantations ending in mealy-mouthed conclusions that merely repeat what's already been said in the body of the articles.[23]

The incentive for contributing to medical literature, I suppose, is that in the future, people might misrepresent footnotes from your obsolete article—and so it goes, as Kurt Vonnegut said.[24]

A Few Last Words, Referenced

In conclusion, people say that footnotes are like a long telephone game that can be traced to early tribes, and that the primal original source material that began the whole chain letter that we call footnotes was found in the early Tarzan movies when Tarzan yelled something along the lines of "Um-gow-wah,"[25] and every animal on Hollywood and Vine came running into the sound studio obediently, like writers.

References

The author states that his dog ate his footnotes.

THE UGLY SIDE OF PEER REVIEW

Jules M. Rothstein, PhD, PT, FAPTA

Views on peer review are a lot like perspectives on surgery. Opinions on the pain associated with the procedure are a function of whether you are doing the cutting or being cut. Unfortunately, or I suppose fortunately from the surgeon's point of view, wielders of scalpels cannot be forced for the purposes of developing empathy to undergo every procedure they conduct (or at least not until we make some more progress in virtual reality). Surgeons, unlike peer reviewers, are forced to forego real-life experiences in favor of imagining the results of their efforts.

Peer reviewers on the other hand become peer reviewers only after they have been on the receiving end of the process, and most reviewers continue to publish and experience the process as recipients of reviews even as they review the works of others. If you think that means we always find the process acceptable and view it with the cool logic of seasoned scientists, you had better think again!

Peer review is a messy process, and it produces more angst than an Ingmar Bergman movie. Unfortunately, I know of no acceptable substitute for the peer-review process. My reactions to rejection and feedback are just like those of other authors who submit manuscripts for publication, reactions that I think are almost universal. Perhaps the human genome codes for reactions to peer reviews (whether they are reviews of articles, grants, clinical practice, or job performance), and there appears to be precious little genetic diversity here. The sequence begins with an immediate reaction of hurt, which progresses to anger born out of frustration. Sometimes you speed through the first phase so quickly you never knew you were hurt because anger becomes so dominant.

You are seized by the notion that the fools offering you suggestions (1) did not understand what you wrote; (2) spent too little time examining relevant issues; (3) were confused by their own biases; and (4) came from uncertain parentage and know little of research, practice, or whatever else they were supposed to be reviewing. These observations are accompanied by a barely repressible desire to set a new world distance record using the reviewer's comments as a Frisbee, or to see if those inflammatory comments could be used as kindling.

Fortunately, this passionate phase during which denial abounds is often followed by bargaining. We selectively see value in some comments so that we may rationalize the fury that remains over remarks that we believe really miss the point. In this manner, we give our own views a mantle of credibility. Because we act as if we have given ground, we assume we must be bringing a reasoned view to our analyses. Unfortunately, this bargaining is usually a ploy to keep us from really looking at the comments with a dispassionate eye. Calm reflection comes only after a period of cooling down, the duration of which differs greatly based on our personalities, our need to see our paper published, or the degree to which we took the comments personally.

We know that we are not supposed to take the comments personally and good peer reviews should be written in a nonpersonalized manner, but who are we kidding? When we have put our life's blood into our efforts, we find it hard to disentangle our egos and identities from our work. But eventually we must do this and, make no mistake, that is neither easy nor something that comes without experience. People who see an article as their only potential publication are more likely to feel pain and experience fury than those who can look at an effort along a continuum and know that the next paper will be better. Imagine treating only one patient in a lifetime and failing to help that patient!

Some people never progress to the last phase because they throw their papers and the comments in

---

Reprinted from Physical Therapy, © 1995; 75(7):582–584, with the permission of the APTA. Edited from the original.

a drawer where they lie as silent monuments to apparent failure and very real frustration. This is a tragedy, because the last reaction is reasoned acceptance. During this phase you not only find that you agree with many of the comments, you are even embarrassed because you missed some mistakes. You still may, however, find areas of disagreement with the reviewers, but such contentions are now based on analysis rather than emotion. You no longer question the parentage of the reviewers, and you even may grudgingly admit that they have given you fodder for thought and ideas for this or other papers. There usually remains some lingering resentment, the kind of resentment we reserve for those who have told us what we needed to hear but did not want to hear.

During this final stage we cannot deny that no matter how much we liked or disliked the reviews, they resulted in our reevaluating our own work. Through reevaluation we grow and garner insights, even if we do little more than develop arguments to counter the comments of the reviewers. While this may not always bring peace, it does lead toward resolution and constructive actions that may make an existing paper better or a future work more credible and clear. I feel bad for those who do not come to this final stage and hope that more people will work through the tangle of emotions that too often keeps them from reconciling their views with the feedback they have been given. When authors fail to respond to reviewers, the process seems more like an inquisition than the source of new knowledge.

I am haunted by this thing we call peer review and never cease wondering how it can be improved. Even after personally writing more than 1,600 letters to authors, I still approach each letter feeling a heavy burden. Just as every person is someone's child, so is each manuscript someone's "child" and I attempt to treat it with respect and care. But the peer-review process requires candid remarks, and in the end decisions must be made. The reality of those remarks and the need for honest feedback deny us the opportunity to sugarcoat and to offer disingenuous and responsibility-shirking remarks—even if we wanted to. For those who have been hurt by the process, I offer my heartfelt apologies because the process is designed to refine and improve the author's work and to nurture growth, not just to judge. Any attempts to judge without providing constructive feedback diminish the process, rob authors and readers, and in our case diminish our credibility with a society that trusts us.

Discussions of peer review are often cloaked in such sanctimonious prose that one might think a religion was being described rather than a flawed process by which colleagues evaluate the work and performance of one another. And, as we all know, growth rarely comes without some awkward and often painful moments, moments that we must learn to endure for a greater good.

NICKELS AND DIMES

Leonard Laster

The other day I finally reached the limits to my patience with financial creativity in American industry. As I completed the order form to buy an $8 item from a catalog company, I realized that the charge for shipping and handling, or S&H, was almost 50% of the cost of the item. With this flash of insight, I surveyed some other catalogs piled on our mail table and found that S&H charges range between 25% and 60% of a purchase price. I'm no economist but I would guess that the S&H stealth charge has become a significant factor in the profits of many U.S. corporations. I would also bet that if I brought in my own operations analyst I would find that the S&H charge routinely far exceeds the actual cost of shipping and handling.

Before the government realized that it had outfoxed itself and modified its Medicare reimbursement requirements, industry seized the day and moved briskly to adopt the new nickel-and-dime technique. When the mail order complex developed the S&H ploy, the telephone companies were also quick to learn how to do well by billing for bits and pieces. Now my telephone company imposes separate charges for connecting the telephone wire to my house, for checking the outside line when there is trouble, for checking the inside line when there is trouble, for checking the equipment when there is trouble, for providing directory information (whether it is correct or not), for dialing the number supplied by the directory information service, for providing call-waiting service, and so on. Telephone companies are cleaning up by using the old Medicare approach.

On the other hand, telephone companies have missed several other lucrative opportunities. Now they charge only a single fee when you dial a multi-digit number. Instead, telephone companies could charge a fee for the first three digits dialed and then impose an R-D (Remaining-Digit) fee for each additional digit dialed. The fee for making a call includes both connecting you with the dialed number and allowing you to talk for so much money per minute. Instead, there could be separate fees for dialing, connecting, and conversing. Thus, if you actually want to talk to someone after you've been connected to the number you're dialing, you pay the conversation fee.

Then there is the matter of content. All telephone calls are not created equal. A collect call from your college-student son in urgent need of money for a ticket to a once-in-a-lifetime rock concert should have a higher monetary value than a nonspecific, emotionally neutral call to check whether he passed Societal Issues 101. And neither call has the same monetary value as a call from your aged mother in a distant city who wants to know why it's been more than two weeks since you made the last eight-hour drive for a visit. A sliding-scale charge based on the emotional content of calls could spruce up the balance sheet of any telephone company and pay for its innumerable TV ads.

Appliance dealerships could also extend the range of their itemized charges. Now they only charge for delivering and setting up a TV set and for an insurance policy that guarantees a working set for the next three months. That's small potatoes nickel-and-diming. What about separate fees for seeing a program and for hearing a program? What about differential charges for fuzzy pictures or clear pictures, uplifting evening news or murder-and-mayhem evening news, and even for half-hour periods of silence? Publishers could get into the act by informing you that if you want to read the concluding chapter of the book you just bought, you must send a request to the publisher together with a proof of purchase seal and a check or money order for S&H. My strategy for extending the S&H concept may sound like a throwaway idea, but I caution any company intending to implement it that the concept is fully protected and I expect handsome royalties and other rewards for its use.

Reproduced with permission. HOSPITAL PRACTICE 1998; 33(2):67. © 1998 The McGraw-Hill Companies, Inc. Edited from the original.

I have decided to follow the operating guidelines of successful American industries and to bill companies for my "time and aggravation." I've set an hourly fee for time and graded fees for degrees of aggravation, and the schedule is available for review. Now when I call a health insurance company to inquire why a $170 physician charge for removing a wart has been allowed only a $2 reimbursement and I'm put on hold for 20 minutes and then transferred to another extension where I am put on hold again and eventually disconnected, I will submit a bill for my time and aggravation.

I rank my time and aggravation strategy at a level with another of my ingenious strategies—dealing with the telemarketing calls that flood our household. Whenever a huckstering stranger interrupts dinner to greet me with "Hello Len," and then offers to sell me a fool-proof system for making tons of money, I interrupt to say that I am required by law to explain that our conversation is being recorded for use as evidence in a class action suit for invasion of privacy. Then I say that if he wishes to go on with this presentation, he must provide his name, telephone number, and address for use in the lawsuit. This fully operational system has failed only once to clear the line immediately.

In contrast, my time and aggravation concept needs debugging. One problem revealed itself when a female catalog company representative informed me that the cost for a transaction included an S&H charge that amounted to 35% of the price of my purchase. I responded that during my last encounter with her company they had sent the wrong item, had forced me to go to the trouble of repacking and reshipping the item, and that I now planned to deduct from her price quote my own charge for "T&A." After an ominous pause, she said that I had no right to talk to her so rudely and hung up. I had no idea what had made her so angry until some time later when a young friend explained that in our decadent society "T&A" stands for something other than "Time and Aggravation."

After that setback, I decided to call a temporary truce with American industry while I think up an inoffensive acronym to replace "T&A." When I told my wife that until I did so, we ought to call a halt to all of our catalog purchases and even cut back on other family expenditures in the free-market world, she simply muttered, "So what else is new?" and walked away.

[Readers please note that there are three even more incisive concluding paragraphs in this piece. If you wish to read them, please send your request to the publisher. Don't forget to include a check to cover a $1 charge for the text and a $40 charge for S&H and ELM (Editor's Lunch Money)].

INFORMATION MANAGEMENT TRUTHS IN SMALL BYTES

Bruce A. Friedman, MD

Computers as Work Savers

Physicians buy computers to help them work more efficiently. When the computers arrive, the doctors are too busy working inefficiently to use them.

Laboratory information systems (LIS) are often bought to conserve resources but rarely succeed at doing this. An LIS adds so much value to laboratory information that any potential savings are eliminated in performing new tasks.

The deployment of an LIS shifts manual work from the lab and patient care units to the information system. When the LIS manager seeks to transfer personnel to the LIS to compensate for this shift, all workers are occupied elsewhere, performing other important tasks.

Printed test reports sent to hospital physicians are often incorrectly routed. To guarantee accurate delivery, multiple copies are generated. The extra copies clog distribution channels, making it harder to route reports.

The Price of Information

Before buying a laboratory information system, you will have to analyze lab procedures in order to understand the flow of information well enough to improve it. Then you will no longer need the LIS.

A voluminous and highly detailed request for proposal (RFP) developed in preparation for the purchase of a high-quality LIS may scare away many vendors of such systems from the bidding process.

If the LIS sales representative is having difficulty describing the features of a system and the audience can't understand the presentation, the rep is either trying to communicate or trying *not* to communicate.

Prepare for a formal LIS site visit by showing up the evening before the formal tour and asking night shift personnel how well the system works. They won't defend a dud.

The final stage of negotiation with an LIS vendor is to address unresolved issues. If earlier stages were carried out properly, there shouldn't be any.

Installing and Learning the System

To manage the professional consultant engaged to advise you about your LIS, you'll need to learn so much about the system that you may not need a consultant after all.

When installing an LIS, one-third of lab personnel will accept change, one-third will maintain a "wait-and-see" attitude, and one-third will resist. LIS personnel will work for the first group, with the second, and on the third.

Making all laboratorians active participants in LIS projects minimizes friction. The optimist calls this strategy empowerment; the cynic, co-optation.

It's easier to teach a medical technologist about computers than to teach a computer expert about medical technology.

A hospital information system (HIS) is best managed centrally to improve the quality of system and information management. Such centralization inevitably fails to empower the very personnel who create and use the information, thereby alienating them and precipitating an immediate decline in the quality of hospital information.

When LIS personnel are overworked, the sophisticated manager will quickly assign information management duties to other laboratorians. The manager thus increases the pool of knowledgeable end-users,

---

Reprinted with permission of the author and Medical Laboratory Observer, © 1992; 24(1):52–54. Edited from the original.

who will then place even greater demands for information processing on LIS personnel.

When the staff continually carps about trivial LIS problems, the system must be working well.

Computers and Civilization

Like the scribes of ancient Egypt, advocates of mainframe computing made their language as complex as possible to insure their own job security. Just as the phonetic alphabet turned hieroglyphics into museum pieces, so will end-user computing, distributed systems, and powerful workstations turn mainframe computers into large disk drives.

Turnover among chief information officers in hospitals is so high that it makes one wonder whether CIO stands for Career Is Over.

A human being is an analog processing and storage device with a bandwidth of 50 bits per second. It excels at pattern recognition but is notoriously slow at sequential calculation. Although its future role in generating laboratory information is debatable, a redesign may enable the device to manage the information product of pathology.

The greatest strategic error in HIS design and development has been the assumption that clinical information is a byproduct of billing information and, consequently, that the medical record is a billing tool. No laboratory professional has ever fallen prey to this delusion.

Information is any difference that makes a difference.

The only real disadvantage of organizational innovation as a way to increase the quality and efficiency of the clinical laboratory is that there is no cost associated with it.

CHAINS OF COMMAND

There may have been a small child out there somewhere who once said, "When I grow up, I want to be middle management." For the rest of us though, it wasn't part of some grand plan, but rather a reward for a job well done. However, each move up the bureaucratic food chain means further removal from daily contact with subordinates. What makes for good management anyway? Probably the best one can hope for is managers that understand work demands even as they become more incapable of performing it themselves.

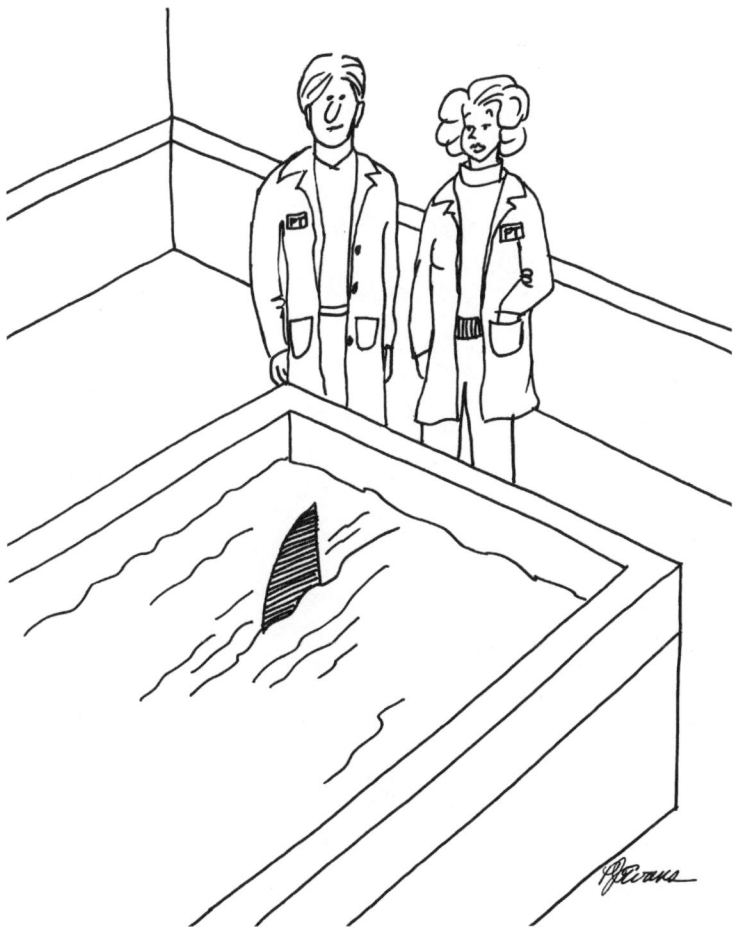

"We find it tends to keep things on schedule."

INTERVIEWERS ARE "LIKE A BOX OF CHOCOLATES"

You Never Know Who You'll Get
Thomas W. O'Connor, PharmD, MBA

Forest Gump's mom was right about life, and the same analogy can be made about interviewers. When you're getting ready for an interview, the possibility of being interviewed by an inexperienced person is the last concern on your mind. However, to quote Forest himself, "it happens," and you need to be prepared.

Before you can deal with inexperienced interviewers, you need to recognize them. They have several common communication traits that quickly give them away.

First, from the outset of the interview, they fail to make you feel at ease. While you're preparing to exchange pleasantries, they're ready to get down to the heart of the matter. Second, they talk more than they listen. Their favorite subjects are usually their company and themselves . . . not necessarily in that order.

Third, their questions, if they ever ask any, represent the extremes in response sizes. Questions either resemble multiple choice on one end of the spectrum or open-book essays on the other. Typical examples of their multiple-choice questions include: "So where are you licensed?" and "When did you graduate?" Their essay-type questions give more opportunity to discuss competencies, but it's hard to know where to begin and end. A favorite essay-type question seems to be: "So, what got you interested in this field of pharmacy and our position specifically?" That's really two questions in one, but combination questions are common too. Finally, inexperienced interviewers will not generally respond to your answer verbally, although you may get an obligatory nod of the head.

Once you've identified the novice interviewer, it's time to deal proactively with this "bad hand." This can be particularly difficult when you're mid-career and find yourself dealing with an early-career novice. Wait for the introductory speech to wind down, and then be prepared to ask the question that you would have most expected. The question should show that you have knowledge of the company. That way you're less likely to receive a second speech usually entitled "who we are."

A good, self-asked, first question might be: "Knowing that your pharmacy is moving in the direction of 'such and such,' let me share my experiences and interests in this area." Now at least you've gained the floor and have a substantive question to answer.

After answering your own question, relinquish the floor to ascertain if the interviewer will now continue in the question-and-answer mode. If not, you'll have to take charge again. If you find that the interviewer is asking either multiple-choice or long essay questions, be prepared to re-word the questions so that they can be answered more fully. Remember that poor questions do not have good answers. Help the interviewer to ask appropriate questions. In essence, you're taking control of the interview, if necessary, to present your qualifications and interests.

For the midcareer interviewee, there are some stumbling blocks that won't score high-interview points. Be careful not to dwell on the past too long. "Remembering when" makes you look like you're not futuristic, and it bores the interviewer. You should also avoid making comparative statements about age, family life cycle, or experience. If what you want to say starts with, "Why, when I was your age . . ." stop to rephrase.

You also need to decide whether to present yourself as a team player or a rugged individual. The

Reprinted with permission from Pharmacy Times, © 1997; 63(5):20.

larger the organization, the more they tend to want team players. The converse is also true. If you assessed a need for a team player, you should discuss your accomplishments in the first-person plural. Using "we" instead of "I" also is less intimidating to the early-career interviewer.

Finally, suggest that you'd be willing to meet with other managers to discuss your potential role in the pharmacy. This gives the inexperienced interviewer a reason to introduce you to others who may take the time to ask additional interview questions informally.

Interviewing is hard enough when you have an experienced interviewer. When preparing for an interview, hope for the best but plan for the worst. One assumption is generally true—you have more at stake than the interviewer so you have probably done more planning for the event. In your planning, remember when and how to conduct your own interview.

THE DAY HELL FROZE OVER IN THE MEDICAL LABORATORY

Michael Ramsey, PhD, MT(ASCP), CLS(NCA)

It had been one of those days every medical technologist dreads. Two techs were out sick, the workload was horrendous, and the chemistry profiler was down. To make matters worse, the phone had rung incessantly since the shift began. At least one tech was tied up answering the phone and looking up some report that the physicians and nurses had ready access to on the floors. Things were backing up, but all the stat orders were being finished and called up within the time limit specified by the medical directors in the laboratory guide.

All of a sudden, Dr. Braxton, an internist, burst through the laboratory door. He headed straight for hematology. Without warning, he confronted Jane B., who was rushing to complete some stat hematology work. Dr. Braxton started shouting obscenities at Jane and accusing her and her co-workers of incompetence and unprofessional behavior for taking so long with his stat request. When Jane tried to ask for the patient's name and the type of tests he requested, her voice was drowned out by more insults.

Finally, the chief pathologist, who had overheard the commotion, entered the hematology department and calmed Dr. Braxton down enough to get the patient's name. At that moment, the ICU nurse walked through the door and told Dr. Braxton that the stat report he had requested had been called up over an hour ago but had been accidentally transcribed onto another patient's chart by the ward clerk. Without saying a word, Dr. Braxton turned and walked out of the laboratory.

Jane, who had similar incidents with other physicians in this hospital, had had enough. She went straight to the head of pathology and turned in her resignation, which was to be effective in two weeks. The laboratory, which was already short-staffed, would be losing one of its best and most experienced techs. We all left the shift that evening with depressing thoughts about our future in this particular laboratory where irate physicians were allowed to insult us in front of our co-workers and where we received no support from the pathologists. Sleep that night did not come easily.

The next morning at work something strange happened. Dr. Braxton came into the laboratory and requested that the chief of pathology ask Jane and everyone present during the altercation the previous day to meet in the laboratory conference room for a few minutes. When we were all present Dr. Braxton began:

Reprinted with permission from Clinical Laboratory Science, © 1994; 7(2):70.

"To begin with, I want to apologize to the tech I shouted at yesterday and to everyone who was offended by my remark. My behavior was immature, inappropriate, and unbecoming of a physician. I acted like a horse's ___ and a jerk. I can only ask for your forgiveness and say that I will strive never to do this again.

My only excuse for my behavior is that I was under tremendous pressure. My patient was very brittle, and I was at a crossroads in his therapeutic regimen. The choice of therapy rested with the laboratory test results which unfortunately had been transcribed onto the wrong chart. The patient is now doing much better, thanks in large part to your work.

Again, I apologize and ask for your forgiveness."

With that, Dr. Braxton left the conference room. We all sat there in total disbelief. Then things really got weird. One of the phlebotomists ran into the conference room to tell us it was snowing outside. This was indeed unusual since it was August and in Louisiana, of all places. On the radio, the weather forecaster said that the most severe blizzard since atmospheric conditions had been recorded was now approaching. The National Weather Bureau could not explain such a phenomenon.

Then I woke up. I sat up in my bed for several minutes trying to interpret what this weird dream meant. Unfortunately, the altercation between Dr. Braxton and Jane had occurred the day before and Jane was leaving our laboratory. Dr. Braxton, however, did not return and no meeting was held in the conference room. So then, what is the meaning of this dream? As far as I can determine, it can mean only one thing.

Almost every medical technologist has experienced the wrath of some tyrannical physician who was allowed to run over hospital policy and other health care professionals' pride. The techs who have other options refuse to put up with such treatment and leave. We somehow expect "short-fused" physicians to apologize when we are "proved innocent" of their accusations. In my experience, this seldom, if ever, happens. The day this type of physician apologizes for insulting a medical technologist or some other health care professional will be "the day that hell freezes over." After all, they do not have a course on manners in medical school!

TEAM BUILDING

Steve Nowak, RT(R), MBA

It was a rather different experience. Instead of stopping by Pandemonium General Hospital to visit with Bill Roentgen, I was headed there to begin my first day working with him. I walked past familiar halls to the proverbial mahogany row. As I opened the door to the suite of executive offices I noticed Bill standing in the back, and started to head in his direction. I was immediately blocked by a young female whose name tag identified her as the Director of Development. Any goalie in the National Hockey League would have been envious of her speed and resolve.

"I'm sorry," she began in a voice that betrayed her statement. "But this area is for administration personnel only!" Bill walked up behind her and put a hand on her shoulder.

"I see you've introduced yourself to your new boss," he said to her, "and made a fine first impression, I'm sure." As we rounded the corner to his office I noticed she was finally able to close her mouth. Bill stepped over to his desk and began sorting through his in box.

"I promised myself that we'd start out on a positive note, so I'm looking for some good news," he began. He continued shuffling papers for several minutes, returned to the top of the stack for a second look, and repeated the routine for a third pass. The ticking of his clock seemed to be getting

Permission granted by Administrative Radiology Journal, © 1998; 17(9–10):28.

significantly louder. Finally, with a look of satisfaction—or mere relief—he pulled a memo from the stack.

"It seems that we've been getting a daily anonymous donation to the hospital auxiliary. It's always coins, comes in a plain brown envelope and has been steady for the past two weeks for a total of $605.88. Not the greatest news in the world, but the small favors add up." There was a knock at the door and after Bill nodded, the hospital's chief of security walked in.

"I hate to bother you, but we've had a character who has been spending every day sitting on the sidewalk in front of the building, begging. I've asked him to leave but he refuses, and wants to speak with you. The police tell me that he is not breaking any laws, so they can't do anything—but he sure makes the place look bad."

"It's a typical Monday," replied Bill and he and I headed toward the hospital's main entrance. After passing through the antique bronze doors we noticed a solitary figure sitting cross-legged on the sidewalk. He was a caricature of the eastern Indian fakir in traditional garb including a turban. A passerby tossed a coin which joined a number of others scattered around him. Bill walked over to him and crouched down so that they were roughly at eye level with one another.

"And how are we today?" began Bill, and the man nodded and smiled. Bill continued, "I must admit that I am curious as to why you're here and what you're doing."

"I am pondering the mysteries of life," replied the man in a very heavy Indian accent. "I am pursuing knowledge and truth." Bill just looked at the man with amused interest.

"For example, I am wondering why in a world which uses computers to reduce paperwork, we instead print more copies of everything that we have recorded in the computers. I am wondering why the people who work in hospitals all wear photographic identification cards except the physicians: I could create much more mischief in a hospital if I were to pass myself off as a doctor rather than a dietary employee."

"Why do doctors, who earn the most money in healthcare, expect free meals and professional discounts for everything from healthcare to theater tickets? Are hospitals a business or a service to the community? I have been contemplating many such questions."

"I see," replied Bill, "and what has prepared you to undertake such a philosophical quest?"

"I have tried to learn from life's experiences so that I might obtain wisdom in such matters," the man replied and Bill rolled his eyes slightly.

"I have also studied at several universities," the man quickly added, "because wisdom also requires a firm rooting in knowledge."

"I see, and what is the most difficult question that you are pondering?" asked Bill as he started to stand.

"Oh that is easy," the man replied, his thick accent disappearing. "I wonder why, with a bachelor's and a master's degree in finance, after sending, faxing, e-mailing and personally delivering copies of my resume, I cannot get an opportunity to interview in your hospital."

"For what it's worth, our Human Resource people have never sent a copy to me." The man reached behind himself and handed a manila envelope to Bill.

"I suspected as much," the man replied. "Fortunately, although my business degrees didn't get your attention, my minor in theater was able to." Bill removed the resume from the envelope and skimmed over its content.

"Impressive," he began. "I'm pleased to meet you, Adam. I think we can talk better inside." Bill extended his hand, but Adam kept Bill waiting while he gathered three dollars and eleven cents worth of coins from the pavement and placed them into an envelope.

"I just need to drop this off with the volunteer from the Hospital Auxiliary at the front desk," he explained. "This will be a total of six hundred eight dollars and ninety-nine cents." He accepted Bill's offered hand and stood up. Bill turned toward me.

"Only a finance person would keep a running total to the penny."

Chains of Command

HOW TO READ A COLLECTIVE BARGAINING CONTRACT:

The Lighter Side of the Management View

Joan Geetter

A collective bargaining contract is like a racing form or a symphonic score. If you can decipher the code, the information is usually clear, if not pleasant. On the other hand, unless you master the key, you are reduced to holding the thing in your hands and making clucking noises, hoping your response passes for the real thing.

Learning what to look for in a few crucial articles will quickly enable you to get the feel of a particular contract. The language in these areas will reveal how the balance of power is tipped, although a word of caution is in order. Like a marriage license, the collective bargaining contract between the parties is no key to the temperature of the relationship. As we all know, people get along well or poorly notwithstanding what is written on a piece of paper. My purpose here is to inform the casual reader where to poke his or her nose to find out who, at least on paper, controls what.

Recognition Clause

In order not to be put off, it is well to think of it as though it were a chapter in Leviticus—something practical but not glamorous. The recognition clause is usually a list, often long and detailed, of who is covered by the agreement. For the writer, its very tedium has special dangers, because proofreadings notoriously fail to catch omissions, which may have unpleasant consequences later on. The purpose of the recognition article is to tell the reader who is in and out of the bargaining unit. In turn, the dividing line between these categories will outline the political configuration of the organization.

To put it simply, before reading any other article in a contract, look at the recognition clause to see to whom it refers. There is little sense in learning the customs of the wrong country.

Board Prerogatives

The next most important article of the agreement to read is the board prerogatives, or as it is called in industry, the management rights section. Also rather tedious, it too is vitally important in that it sets forth the powers of those who run the organization. As a representative of management, I distinguish two basic kinds of management rights clauses: the "putter in" and the "leaver out" varieties. A clause written under the first of these lists every conceivable right, whether exercised or not, that management might want to exercise and sets it down as the sole responsibility or prerogative of management. A clause written under the other variety, which operates on the theory of "unless I have explicitly given it to you, it's still mine," reserves to management everything not explicitly relinquished under some article of the contract. I have written both kinds in contracts, and to tell the truth, it is still too early to tell for certain which is better.

Grievance Procedures

For all practical purposes the grievance procedure is the heart, or perhaps more appropriately, the stomach, of the contract. Next to salary provisions, it is the article with which employees will be most familiar; it will often be the article by which they are introduced to the contract. Whatever popularity the salary article has will be short-lived, while the grievance machinery, like the family stove, gets used over and over. On it, something is always cooking.

Reprinted with permission from Journal of Allied Health, © 1982; 11(3):176–179. Edited from the original.

The first thing to read in a grievance article is the definition section. It will tell you what a grievance is within the meaning of *this* contract. Naive readers assume that a grievance in a contract means what it does in ordinary parlance. That is usually not so. In other words, a grievance is not simply a word for what makes the employee unhappy. It is to his or her peril that an impatient user neglects to discover what restrictions the grievance must conform to before the grievance is eligible for consideration within a particular contract. Here are two examples, one narrow and one broad, of what I'm talking about.

Narrow definition of a grievance: The term grievance shall mean a dispute concerning the interpretation or application of the terms or provisions of this agreement.

Broad definition of a grievance: A grievance means any act, condition, regulation, article of the agreement, or process that the employee believes is unfair to him.

As you can see, under the second definition almost anything the employee believes is unfair (his life, her parking space) is fair game to grieve under the contract. That means the complaint will be championed by the union and perhaps brought before an arbitrator for resolution. Institutions that live under such broad definitions and that also permit binding arbitration on the substance of all these complaints will find that, in effect, their board, and to some extent their administrative structures, have been superseded by the process of arbitration.

Grievance or Complaint?

Time limits explain the difference between a grievance and a complaint. For life to be livable under a contract, it is vitally important to have time limits assigned to what is grievable. Without them the game has no meaning at all. Just as the essence of baseball is to accomplish something within nine innings, so too under a contract the grievant must come forward by a certain date. Time limits, like a death sentence, as Dr. Johnson remarked, concentrate the mind wonderfully.

Still another area to check when reading grievance procedures is whether the procedure permits the grievant to adjust his or her complaint in more than one place simultaneously. Can he or she seek remedies from the Human Rights Commission and the contract at the same time? If so, it may be wise to try to get some informal agreement with the union to permit exhausting one remedy before embarking on another. To those who would avoid this problem, I suggest contract language that permits the employer to drop a grievance when the employee starts up the same battle on another front.

The last and most important segment of a grievance article tells you what final step is available to the grievant. Is the final step outside arbitration by a third party? Is the arbitration binding or advisory? Is arbitration confined to procedural questions, or may the arbitrator deal with a substance of the issue as well? These are important matters. They also relate back to the definition of a grievance mentioned earlier. An unrestricted definition of a grievance may be tolerable, even preferred, if the final step in the grievance process is the board of trustees or the president. On the other hand, if a final decision is to be made by a third party unfamiliar with life at East Cupcake University, then a restricted definition of a grievance is probably best on so-called governance issues.

Footnotes for the Devil's Disciples

1. If you want to have a heyday with your grievance procedure, put in an academic freedom article and make it grievable. That way you can grieve anything at any time as a violation of academic freedom.

2. Don't mention that you prorate salaries for your part-time employees. You may not win ultimately, but you'll have a lot of fun trying to win full payments for half-time employees.

3. Don't limit the salary settlement to those still on the payroll. That way you can pay all of the coaches who have already left town.

THE IMPORTANCE OF BEING LIKE ERNEST

Sanjiva Wijesinha

I well know what a dangerous effect hard work has on the gastric mucosa.

One of my old friends—a 'manager' who consumed cartons of cigarettes and reams of stationery with equal profligacy—recently suffered a massive bleed from his peptic ulcer.

This sobering revelation took my mind back to the time when, years ago, I worked in an institution where the only 'manager' (if one could dignify his job with such a title) was a chap by the name of Sergeant Ernest Mann.

The man had joined the army long before I'd seen my first cadaver and by the time our paths crossed, he was the non-commissioned officer in charge of the medical centre in the one-horse army detachment to which I, as a young Captain in the Army Medical Corps, was posted. It was only a minor medical facility in the Army's vast establishment, but Sergeant Mann ran it with supreme efficiency aided by a well-deserved reputation for taking his time.

He was never seen to hurry.

He never seemed to worry.

He never, as far as I know, lost his temper.

Of course it must be admitted, there were some who claimed that he had never been known to do a full day's work either.

The Masterly Art of Inactivity

Now, during my long medical career, in diverse parts of the world, I have seen plenty of folk who did nothing—but most of the time they would attempt valiantly to create the impression that they were, in fact, busy doing something.

Sergeant Mann, on the other hand, was the only person I know, who was perfectly satisfied, when he was doing nothing, to look as if that is exactly what he was doing.

Reprinted from Australian Family Physician, © 1998; 27(11):1061, with permission of the author.

In the morning, when I turned up for duty at the medical centre, he would greet me with a regulation salute and crisp "Good morning, Sir." Having arranged files on my table, he would then go outside the consultation room, inform the waiting patients in what order they were to go in and then retire to his cubicle to await further orders.

If the phone rang, he answered it. If someone came to him with a query, he dealt with it, using the minimum number of words necessary. He never pretended to busy himself with files or letters or paperclips. He just sat impassively at his desk until he was called.

One significant feature about his style of management was that he never went out of his way to do a job that he felt could be delegated to someone else. At the same time, he never tried to make a decision about a matter which he rightly felt should be resolved by the medical officer.

Those matters which he in his wisdom felt were his to tackle were attended to with minimum fuss and minimum time, after which he reverted to his customary "standby mode."

In short, he was the perfect administrator. He did his job, he let his superiors and subordinates get on with theirs and we all got on with no problems, no complaints and no overspending of budgets.

Managing Busi-ness

Since those far-off days, I have worked in a variety of medical institutions, each equipped with a manager who was eminently more qualified and better paid than my lowly sergeant.

Most of these important individuals were so busy performing a plethora of tasks to justify their existence that I have longed for the days when Sergeant Mann was content to do his allotted task and let those about him get on with theirs.

Mann was a man who knew his job and didn't feel it necessary to create a flurry of activity and a ream of paperwork to prove to the outside world that he was performing his duties.

Perhaps Sergeant Mann's technique of masterly inactivity was applicable only to the kind of small practice we had at the time. It may be that there is some truth in the assertion that as numbers multiply and technology advances, medical establishments need hyperactive managers to efficaciously utilise the resources of the 1990s. I sometimes wonder. Sergeant Mann, as far as I knew, never had problems with heartburn or peptic ulcers.

When I last heard from him, he was retired from the Army, alive and well and enjoying in earnest a life of grandmasterly inactivity.

A CHILLING TALE

Sirenhead

Dear Sirenhead: Our communications center supervisor informed us of a situation reportedly happening around the country. I think it is a bunch of bunk, so I figured I would go to the source of all true knowledge: Sirenhead.

This supervisor received an e-mail from the EMS coordinator of one of our local fire departments. It advised that someone or some group has targeted traveling salesmen for kidney removal after slipping them a mickey in a bar. Supposedly, when the "patient" wakes up, he finds himself in a bathtub filled with ice and has a note and a phone next to him. The note advises the patient to "Call 9-1-1 or you will die." The patient then discovers two 9-inch slits on his lower back, where the kidneys were removed. Sometimes, there's an IV running.

Has the esteemed Sirenhead or his sources heard of this? Is this another example of false information traveling around the country via e-mail and word of mouth? Many of my fellow employees believe this story, so I told them I would check with a couple of sources.

— B. Smith via Internet

I do have the scoop on this. The victims aren't salesmen, they're traveling aerobics instructors who, after being on their feet all day, go back to their hotel, order room service and slip into a hot bath to soak their tired feet. A deranged anorexic crippled by one too many high-impact sessions lies in wait as room service arrives. On the way in, the delivery dude always leaves that stupid little latch near the top of the door in the way so the door doesn't close behind him. So this sicko places an EKG electrode over the lock plate, preventing the door from locking as the delivery guy leaves the room. Our maniac waits, slips in, performs the operation and leaves.

The part that has detectives intrigued is how the perpetrator performs the major operation so quickly. The leading theory proposes that they have trained a mysterious creature called a snipe to abet in this horrendous crime. Because snipes are nocturnal, they can stealthily harvest the victim's organs under the cover of darkness.

OK, let's grope our way back to reality. You and your pals are entrusted with saving lives every day. You're well trained and experienced. I'll bet you've seen people die from everything from a rectal bleed to a nosebleed. It doesn't take much to bleed to death from an unattended wound. If someone slit you open (twice), took out both your kidneys (duh!) and left you in the tub (ice or no ice), you'd die. How could you fall for this crap? This is just another story zooming throughout cyberspace to lots of gullible eyes.

Please bring your pals down to reality and tell Captain Kirk at the Comm Center to chill!

P.S. Know anyone interested in a slightly used spleen?

Reprinted with permission from JEMS: Journal of Emergency Medical Services, © 1998; 23(7):96.

REENGINEERING FOR THE BIRDS

Darlene Sredl

Large institutions are routinely troubled by well-meaning, though weak-bladdered, members of the Avian community. Sometimes, however, the institution itself is for the birds. Such is the case as we look in on Metropolis Health Center, just down the street from market-share rival, Our Lady of Perpetual Payment. We have a bird's eye view as they flock to the Hospital bored room, conveniently branched off the Administrative Roost.

It was obvious that the CEO did not want to go out on a limb by himself, or possibly lay an egg; so, he called the brood together to incubate the seed of a bold new Vulture—reengineering. The meeting began with some Flamingo dancers for light entertainment. "Call the Role. Where's your pen, Gwen?"

"Right here sir, ready to take down every word."

The pecking order included:

Robin Nightingale—Director of Nestlings
The Ruffled Grouse—Assistant Director of Nestlings
The Yellow-Bellied Sapsucker—V.P. (Operations)
The Humming Bird—Chief Financial Officer (CFO)
The Balding Corporate Legal Eagle
The Common Snipe—Director of Security
The Southern Dodo—Director of Maintenance
The Albino Peacock—Director of Housekeeping
The Cockatoo—Assistant Director of Housekeeping
The Bare-Faced Buzzard—Director of Marketing
The Red-Necked Loon—Director of Psychiatry
And, of course, in the Captain's Nest, the Horn-Rimmed Owl, as CEO

The obfuscation began, "We are gathered together today to talk about reengineering and the new economic enterprise."

"You mean, Trekkies?" queried the CFO.

"The CFO must have seen a UFO!" quipped the Buzzard.

"Reengineering is the new buzzword, Buzzard. We're talking about our new adversarial competitive strategy. First, we map out a framework for change and then we allocate appropriate resources to accomplish that change. Let's hear it from the Vice President. Which vice are you presiding over today?"

"Gift shop lottery sales are way off."

"Why?"

"I think somewhere in our employee manual it says you can't gamble while on duty."

"Hum-m-m..." mused the CFO. "To gambol means to walk around casually and with no definite purpose, doesn't it?"

"Yes sir!"

"Well, that describes most of our employees," ruffled the Grouse.

"OK, so we will continue to prohibit loitering or casual walking. We will continue to prohibit gamboling on company time. The secretary just has to chickenscratch a few letters in the manual. No major rewrite. Now, back to the lottery sales—I want the gift shop profits up!"

"Why not let the employees use their I.D. badge like credit cards to make purchases?" suggested the Dodo.

"Oh, no, Dodo, are you suggesting we put it on their bills? Humm-m-m..." mused the Humming Bird.

"What multi-skilled pluralistic thinking. What statistical congruence! That is the seed of a great idea!" screeched the owl. "Quack. Get it signed and witnessed by a Notary Republic."

"I think Democrats should have an equal say. After all, this is an election year"... mused the Wren.

"Figures for high performance employee resources must be bottomed out," the CFO continued.

"How are we going to do that?" challenged the Mocking Bird. "How are we going to find the personnel? The type of employee we seek is not going to work for chickenfeed."

Reprinted with permission from Journal of Irreproducible Results, © 1998; 43(1):16–17.

"How do you screen potential new employees?" asked the CEO.

"Security runs a record chick. Many are afowl of the law. Some come straight from the pen," snipped the Snipe.

"Then," concluded the CFO, "Hire only jailbirds."

"What?"

"You said they're willing to work for scratch, didn't you? Besides, you could put peepers in their pockets so we would know where they are in case they're thinking of flying south and, we can buy their uniforms from Amber Crowbee and Finch."

"The Hell I can."

"What did you say?"

"The Pelican, we need a Pelican on our bored to oversea them."

"Remember," added the CEO, "fragmented operations focus functional barriers to the integrated processing systems that have downgraded this hospital's consumer applications."

"What does that mean, sir?" they cried in unison.

"My little chickadees, it means that the healthcare consumer is integral but unnecessary. Furthermore, the infrastructure we used to rely on can no longer empower or subjugate a breakdown in the chassis system so that the logarithm of success is as farfetched as ever. Are you all birdbrains?"

"Oh, thank you for explaining it sir," cheaped the CFO.

"Validation and construct integrity continue to dominate our vision," the CEO raled on.

"Do you need glasses, Sir?"

"Horn rims, remember?"

"Let's consider the platform alternatives," continued the CEO.

"Running for President, Mr. President?"

"I'm talking about *artificial* intelligence."

"We've used that for years."

"I mean *Real* artificial intelligence."

"We prefer Apple Computers for the obvious reason, of course."

"Outsource foodsource?"

"Yeah, Birdseye products."

"But, I deduced . . ."

"You could get arrested for that, sir," the Snipe interjected.

"But, the proposition must touch everyone . . ."

"There you go again, Mr. President." The Grouse's feathers ruffled.

"Don't you want to see the new digital system?" he asked the Ravenfeathered Nightingale.

"Not NOW, sir!"

"Spreadsheet?"

"Innuendo!"

"You would peck'er?"

"I object" thundered the legal eagle.

"On what grounds?"

"Habeus Corpus Luteum."

"Oh, Ok, OK. Back to the basics. Anticipate, initiate, precipitate. We cannot Parrot the past. That's a Cardinal sin. The key challenge? Abstractions and contradictions. Our minds must be open to any possibility including impossibility. I say, the values of this organization shall remain firm unless they become dispensable," the CEO warbled on.

"We can begin an excremental improvement program," offered the Director of Avian Resources.

"Hey, cleaning is my territory," squawked the Peacock.

"Preening, not cleaning is your territory," countered the Mocking Bird who continued, "For example, sabbaticals. We could give employees three months off every seven years."

"But, current market research indicates the average avian lifespan just approaches 5.8 years."

"Exactly! We won't have to EsCrow any retirement. What a savings," squawked the CFO.

"In conclusion, we must forge ahead with corporate competency and myopic instability. Overall, never remember to forget. We must end what we have begun and begin what must end. Teamwork will boldly rebuild the framework of the future and converge upon an axis of revolution. I say, Healthcare must . . . not only molt, it must revolt . . ."

"Sir. It's already revolting!"

THE INDESTRUCTIBLE *BACILLUS BUREAUCRATICUS*

Robert M. Goldwyn, MD

Description

Bacillus bureaucraticus, subspecies of *Homo sapiens*, genus Homo (man): a two-legged organism, worldwide distribution, reproduces exponentially, epidemic and pandemic, identifiable by characteristic pose: seated, with pencil in one hand and telephone in the other; secretes methylcellulose sheets (paper) used for both defense and offense to suffocate enemies, obtains nutrition from others.

History

Appears very early in human records; first description in caves, with portrayals of hunting: one hunter and clump of *Bacillus bureaucraticus* in background. Various other descriptions of this organism can be found throughout the centuries:

Petronius (died A.D. 66): ". . . I was to learn later in life that we tend to meet any new situation by reorganizing . . . and a wonderful method it can be for creating the illusion of progress while producing inefficiency and demoralization."

Honoré de Balzac (1799–1850): "Bureaucracy is a giant mechanism operated by Pygmies."

General Sir Walter Walker (in 1981): "Britain has invented a new missile. It's called the Civil Servant—it doesn't work and it can't be fired."

Two encounters in one day gave me further information, if any were needed or wanted, into the pathophysiology of the *Bacillus bureaucraticus*. The first was an article I happened to read. It concerned cataract surgery and the possible abuses through Medicare. Its gist was that "during the first 9 months of 1989, Medicare spent $980,000 to deny $42,000 worth of cataract operations." Not included in this doleful statement was the number of person hours devoted to the search for felons. Was it worth it? Yes, in theory; possibly yes, in actuality. After all, the pursuit of those who perpetrate fraud or theft or murder is always expensive, yet the effort is necessary in the hope not only to catch the criminal, but to prevent greater illegality. Nevertheless, the data concerning cataract operations are sobering: almost $1 million spent for a yield of about one-fiftieth that amount.

My second encounter with the sinister and ubiquitous *Bacillus bureaucraticus* was in connection with my reapplying to a hospital staff. That process, I am convinced, has been made purposefully tedious to discourage the casual applicant; it now almost turns away the worthy and once-enthusiastic applicant.

The staff registrar had returned my application because I had not had photocopies of my certificates from the American Board of Surgery and the American Board of Plastic Surgery notarized. My oversight initiated a search at the hospital for a Notary Public (why do we not say a "Public Notary"?). After numerous inquiries, including at least five telephone calls, I located one, whose office I entered. After having stated my need to the Notary's secretary, who, though small in stature, was gigantic in obstructionism, I received the following response:

"Ha," he croaked, "I wish we could help you, Doctor, but Mr. ___, who does the notarizing, is working on the budget all this week. He couldn't possibly take care of you. He is using every minute of his time."

That description alone made me want to see his boss, who must be a marvel—the first human being to be continuously and completely productive.

"But," I was about to say, when I noticed that the secretary had returned to his typewriter, undoubtedly generating another classic piece of literature—a directive that at once would eradicate a disease and quadruple the hospital's endowment.

Reprinted with permission from Plastic and Reconstructive Surgery, © 1991; 87(1):139–141. Edited from the original.

While not being as prescient as Nostradamus or as insightful as Freud, I, nevertheless, recognized that further words from me would have been futile. The secretary's mind had closed like a microclamp. I knew I would never pierce the radar screen guarding that mighty cortex. As I stumbled from the office, I realized that bureaucrats are masters and mistresses of inflexibility.

To lessen reader anxiety, I should state that I finally found within the hospital a Notary, who was typing. At first she asked me to return in a day or two. By this time, like a man crazed from thirst in the desert, I begged her for the "holy seal." Being merciful, she consented and devoted the next 2½ minutes of her extremely valuable time to executing the document.

I confess that for a few minutes that day I worried about my cerebral control. Would I be able to withstand what was obviously a plot against me? Was I being singled out for the kill, like each of General Custer's scouts? Fortunately, I realized that this would be impossible: bureaucracy could never think that effectively or creatively. No, this was simply an observation I had made about a disease that is so pandemic that it has become almost unrecognizable. What we feared would happen to medicine has now come to pass. To get anything done nowadays requires infinite fortitude and foreplay.

The proliferation of extramedical personnel to manage medicine is a comparatively recent phenomenon. We doctors thought that we were immune to the *Bacillus bureaucraticus*, that bureaucrats and regulations were for others. How foolish of us! Today, medicine has created or has had created for it a third state that is supposedly working for the benefit of the patient primarily. If one believes this, one will believe anything. The primary group that bureaucrats serve is themselves. In this endeavor, they are without peers. Corporate mentality and consensus judgment have replaced the individualism that once characterized physicians and the profession. Personal accountability, the basis of any relationship between two human beings, is almost out of style, as rare as an Air Force general wearing an Elizabethan collar.

A piece in *Modern Heath Care*, which is, in its own words, "the business news magazine for health care management," confirmed my impressions of what each of us is likely witnessing in our hospitals. The cover title of the story alone is sufficient to get the message: "Hospital Bureaucracy: A Story that Answers the Question: How Many Managers Does It Take to Screw up a Change of Light Bulbs?" Too many. Many hospital executives are beginning to recognize that "overly complex organizational structures have increased their costs without any corresponding financial or service benefits." One administrator candidly noted: "We placed too much emphasis on process. It was part cultural and part leadership style. We got everyone involved, but it impeded decision making." Evidently, under cost-based reimbursement, particularly under Medicare, hospitals recovered more money if they broke down costs into several components, thereby increasing the total charges. The article cited respiratory therapy as an example. It was once performed by nurses. A hospital managing consultant observed that "if cost-based reimbursement continues, we'd probably see hospitals break out 'enema therapy' next."

Another factor leading to needless layers of management is the hospital chief executive officers themselves. "With little or no concern over cost increases, CEOs (chief executive officers) added people to solve management problems and a lot of managers built their own substructures." It might be said of this situation that never before have so many people done so little for so many.

I am not a totally irrational optimist, although I happen to be a surgeon. Even I realize that this editorial is my alternative to tranquilizers and psychoanalysis. I have neither the inclination for the former nor the time for the latter. I do fear, however, what is likely to happen when a person in need rushes into the hospital and asks "Is there a doctor here?" The response will probably be: "Yes, we do have one on display—in the museum. He [or she] died of infection from *Bacillus bureaucraticus*. To get there—to the museum—take your first right up the stairs, your third left down the corridor, go through the glass doors—even though you will see a sign saying "Do Not Enter"—following the black line back again into the basement. But, before you go, please fill out this form—in triplicate."

THE ORGANIZATION ZOO: A FABLE

John G. Bruhn, PhD
Alan P. Chesney, PhD

The Fable

One day, the zookeeper was gone. The myna birds, known for picking up words from patrons of the zoo, said, "Let's organize; let's organize." The gorillas beat their chests, the chimps jumped up and down, the lions roared, the hyenas laughed, and the peacocks spread their tail feathers—all signifying approval. The majority of animals were unenthusiastic; the ostrich buried its head; the seals, otters, and sea lions busily raced one another from one end of their pool to the other; the bears slept; the hippos took a mud bath; and the mountain goats ranged, outside of hearing, on the top of the ridge. Since it never requires a majority to get anything started, the minority decided to form an organization. The animals knew they had as much right to be in charge as the zookeeper. If necessary, they could always call upon the Humane Society to protect their rights.

Leader

Who would be the leader? The giraffe, who had the best perspective of the zoo, suggested that an election be held. The zoo's prima donna, the peacock, felt best qualified, the bison felt most experienced, the lion believed he had the "presence" of a chief executive officer (CEO), and the gorilla knew he could intimidate most anyone; but the chimps, who heard all of the campaigning, laughed and jumped up and down, because they knew that in this age of political correctness, the leader would have to be either a black or brown bear. All the animals believed their leader should be a known entity from within their own ranks, not a rare or endangered type, and certainly not a farm animal. The black bear was elected CEO.

Structure

The next issue was the type of organizational structure they would have. They considered the pyramid, but discarded it because the bear's managerial style was to roam around the organization rather than sit at the top. The rectangle was discarded because it required the animals to take sides. The circle was discarded because all of the animals could not get around a table. The animals wanted a futuristic organizational structure. They heard about quality circles from the zoo patrons, and, since patrons were their clients, they listened. The zoo patrons expected quality service; with the diverse ways in which service in the zoo was provided, the animals thought quality circles most closely resembled the type of organization they should have. Quality circles were formed, each with a leader. The gorillas, chimps, orangutans, and all of the water animals formed a quality circle that provided entertainment for the patrons; it was important that these animals liked to perform. The peacocks, lions, elephants, bears, tigers, and hippos formed a quality circle whose service was to appear for photographs. Since most of the animals in this circle liked to sleep, their pose for photographers was always natural. Some animals didn't fit in quality circles with others because they were too ugly (hyena, bison, rhino), too large (giraffe), too remote (mountain goat), too unfriendly (turtle, ostrich), or wouldn't talk to patrons (parrot). These animals were named supervisors and directors.

Organizational Components

Some members of organizations are independent, competitive, and seek individual rewards; new organizational structures that stress teams, quality circles, and task groups make it difficult to satisfy their ego needs. Indeed, the animals in the zoo have a variety of egos. Animals are kept in cages not only to protect the patrons but also to protect the animals from each other's egos. But cages didn't keep the animals from forming an organization, albeit

Adapted with permission from The Health Care Supervisor, © 1996; 4(3):13–20, and publisher.

different from the formal organization of which the zookeeper knew he was in charge.

Every organization needs an advisory committee. The animals selected the bison, the oldest and most experienced, to chair the committee. The myna birds and parrots were named to head up public relations and the giraffe, who knew everyone's business, was charged with fund raising. The black bear, as CEO, commanded the full attention of the advisory committee as he laid out goals and objectives for the organization. The advisory committee was to help promote the zoo to patrons, obtain financial support for improvements and the acquisition of new types of animals, and lobby for animal rights. The bear explained that the animals had adopted a mission statement that they would provide the best entertainment, photographic opportunities, and human-sensitive animals of any zoo in the country. Other zoos might be larger, have more exotic animals, or even have a special zoo for children, but this zoo was unique because it tried harder.

The zoo organization seemed to work well. The animals let the zookeeper believe he was in charge, and he was, when it was time to feed the animals and clear out the patrons so everyone could sleep.

Programs

By listening to and watching the patrons, the animals quickly learned important words that would help make the new organization a success: "benchmarking," "diversity," "change management," "pay for performance," and "outplacement" were used frequently to help the animals choose a course of action. Since only the words were learned, they took on new meanings at the zoo.

The black bear created teams that were charged with implementing the new words. The birds were charged with benchmarking. They flew out of the zoo, observed other organizations, and brought back ideas about how to be more productive and how to measure zoo performance. Soon, the bear was measuring popularity to determine which animals were most popular with the patrons and therefore most productive.

The hoofed animals were put in charge of diversity. They studied the variety of animals in the zoo and concluded that certain farm animals should be included. They brought in horses, sheep, cows, and pigs because these animals were underrepresented in the zoo population. Although they did not contribute to the photographic or entertainment value of the zoo, it was hoped that, in time, these animals would learn how they could contribute.

Because the bear, as CEO, wanted to introduce change gradually, he chose the reptiles to form a team on change management. The reptiles moved slowly, under cover, and since they were almost noiseless, could surprise the animals with new ideas. Originally, the reptiles resisted change, but they learned from the chameleon, who changed colors to fit its environment, that it was important to please the boss. Soon the reptiles were presenting workshops to the other animals on how to become peak performers. The snakes carefully monitored change so that whatever changes occurred, their own niche in the organization was not threatened.

One day, the water animals, sea lions, seals, otters, and dolphins approached the bear with a new concept called "pay for performance." The idea was to distribute the organization's scarce resources to the animals on the basis of the value of each animal's contribution to the organization's goals. The logic of this system, with its emphasis on rewarding those animals who were most important to the organization's success, led to a new and improved reward system, which was designed to motivate the animals to be more productive. The water animals, who were both entertaining and photogenic, benefited greatly from the new plan. Unfortunately, the elephants, hippos, and rhinos, who had a greater need for rewards (food), found that they were getting less and less.

All of these changes meant that some of the animals were not needed for the efficient operation of a first-class zoo. The bear, therefore, needed to develop an outplacement program. The big cats were placed in charge of this function. The tigers, lions, jaguars, and cougars, being hunters, were able to get rid of dead wood in two ways. The small animals disappeared at night without a trace. The larger animals—the old bison, the elephants, hippos, and rhinos—were outplaced by being sold to circuses.

Problems

The zoo was running very efficiently. The programs had been fully implemented, and the zoo was gaining a national reputation. People came from all over the country to see the model zoo run by the animals. But the new zoo was not without problems.

Basically, there were two problems, which the bear and those who reported to him considered minor. First, the humans who worked at the zoo were getting tired of doing all of the scut work, such as feeding the animals and cleaning the cages. Second, the level of distrust and lack of respect among the animals was increasing. Everyone was fearful of the big cats; if they were seen in your area you might be the next candidate for outplacement. Many animals were jealous of the sea lions, otters, and dolphins, who had the most glamorous jobs and the best pay. Most of the zoo animals distrusted the reptiles who changed opinions as the need arose. No one liked the new farm animals, who were common, or the cleft-hoofed animals, such as the bison, giraffe, gazelle, and antelope, who were perceived to be strong supporters of their farm cousins. Because the birds, led by the owls, hawks, and eagles, were always away from the zoo, looking for prey and conducting studies, the other animals could reach them only by carrier pigeon.

Change and Challenge

The black bear gained national attention as a CEO. He had many speaking engagements and traveled frequently but failed to delegate authority to his line officers when he was gone. The black bear received many awards for being successful in getting the organization established. The President of the United States named him Animal of the Year, and the Humane Society put his picture on their poster. As the zoo flourished, the bear felt that he had met his goals as a CEO. Therefore, he began to look around for his next career opportunity. He wanted to be Commissioner of Wildlife, but no black bear had ever held such a high-level government job. Instead, he was recruited by the San Diego Zoo to be chair of the Zoo Board. This job would give him exposure working with zoos throughout the world, recruiting outstanding and unique animals to San Diego. The San Diego Zoo also had a bachelorette black bear who was looking for a mate. The snake, who overheard the bear's telephone conversation about the job offer with the San Diego Zoo, spread a rumor that the bear was leaving.

The Zoo Board decided the new CEO must be a female, because no female had ever been CEO in the zoo. A dolphin was elected because of her superb ability to communicate with two- and four-legged animals as well as her balanced philosophy of work and play. The dolphin named more sea animals to positions because she believed they had been underrepresented in zoo bureaucracies. Almost immediately, the reptiles began to spread rumors of sexism and favoritism. The myna birds said, "Here we go again; here we go again." The gorillas beat their chests, the chimps jumped up and down, the lions roared, the hyenas laughed, and the peacocks spread their tail feathers. They all knew the moral of this fable: "The more things change, the more they stay the same."

HOW TO ENJOY BEING A CHAIR

Anne Parry, PhD, MCSP, DipTP

Does it choke you to call the person chairing a meeting 'chair'? Do you think it is absurd that all questions should be addressed to a seat with a back and four legs? Do you snarl at another example of 'political correctness'? Do you blench at the sound of 'chairperson'—still worse, 'chairpersonship'? Untie your tongues and recover homeostasis, help is at hand!

The *Oxford Dictionary of New Words* (1991) lists 'chair' as a usage arising from the Feminist movement of the 1970s but says that impersonal use has existed for centuries and provides the precedent.

Reprinted with permission from Physiotherapy, © 1993; 79(12):824.

True, the preoccupation with the etymology of words, in particular the confused and confusing use of "man" to mean both male person and the whole species, caused the appearance of chairpersons (and spokespersons but not policepersons or seapersons).

However, although chairperson got shortened to chair, it is not the late 20th century neutered euphemism it appears to be.

Turn to the *Oxford English Dictionary* (1989) for the history. It dates back to 1658, at least, from when Clarendon is quoted: "The chair behaves himself like a Busby amongst so many schoolboys." *Himself*, note. Using chair to mean the person or the office is a metonym—the word referring to an attribute is substituted for the thing that is meant: "All hands on deck," for example, or using "crown" to refer to the monarch. Context is all. The hands are not disembodied, a crown does not carry a handbag, and a piece of furniture does not chair a meeting.

Away with the silly "madam chairman" that reeks of Edna Everage. If gender is important, stick with chairman or chairwoman. We can happily and correctly, historically, etymologically and politically, address both men and women as "chair," and they can enjoy it.

WHAT'S IN A NAME?

Michael J. Shaffer, DSc

Not long ago I bumped into a BMET I knew at a local hospital. He had on a white coat with "Clinical Engineer" stitched on the front and looked very medical.

"Snodgrass, I thought you were a technician," said I, pointing to this title.

"Right," said he, "but I think 'clinical engineer' has a better ring to it than 'BMET.' The only problem is no one seems to know what a clinical engineer does. General Hospital and St. Elsewhere don't appear to have one, and they're big hospitals."

I tried again. "Snodgrass, you can't do this; you're not qualified."

"Oh yes I can. I'm a professional. I support and advance patient care in my own way, and I apply my engineering and management skills to health care technology. That's what clinical engineers say they do, and that's what I do."

Sensing I was getting nowhere, I hit him with the $64 question. "You must know this state has a law for engineers saying you can't call yourself an engineer just like that."

Snodgrass had an answer even to that one. "I'm told it doesn't apply," he pointed out. "The state law says nothing in it can affect the practice of another profession—like the medical profession."

I gave up. "What are you going to do next?" I asked.

"Well, I think 'Risk Manager' sounds better, so I'm trying to find out what one does."

"Won't your administrator object?"

"Not at all, he likes my initiative."

Reprinted with permission from Biomedical Instrumentation and Technology, © 1993; 27(6):450–451. Edited from the original.

THE MORE THINGS CHANGE

Unless you've been living under a rock for the last few years, you've experienced a rate of change that is awe-inspiring. There seems to appear daily some new gadget or electronic wizard that performs faster and more efficiently than ever before. It's anyone's guess just how these rapid changes will affect the way we perform job duties in the future. But, some workplace events will likely occur forever because of human nature. It's comforting to realize that no matter how sophisticated the technology, we still have the capacity to make each other laugh.

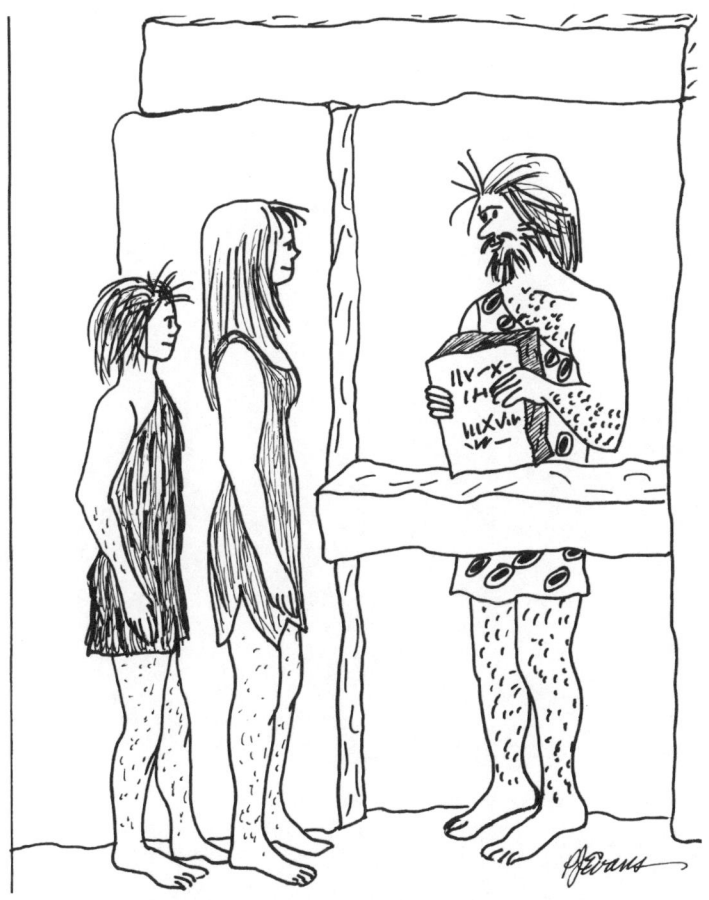

"Your plan covers roots and berries, but not herbs."

MESSAGE TO A GRADUATING CLASS AND NONE SHOULD FAIL

H.F. Helmholz, Jr., MD

Message To A Graduating Class

Remember that you can't remember
Everything we've said,
But you will be some surprised
How much is in your head.
And there's capacity for more,
Learn something every day;
It isn't hard for what you do
Will teach you 'long the way.
When ears and eyes and mind are open
Now you working R.T. creatures
Will earn and learn and pretty soon
You'll know more than your teachers.

None Should Fail

Exams are never easy,
They are not meant to be;
But when you're ready for them,
They're not so bad, you see.
So how can one get ready,
Is there a useful rule?
There really is no ready
Substitute for school.
So having done one's school work,
Why should any flunk?
Maybe your poor teacher
Was handing out the bunk.
But blame the school with care,
'Cause other students pass;
You forgot too much of what
Was handed out in class.
So spend some time in reading,
Don't put your notes away;
Review the little details
You do not use each day.
So if you fail the first time
Seek the remedy
For weaknesses reported by
The NBRC.

Reprinted from Respiratory Care, © 1997; 42(9):848, with permission of the author. Originally appeared in *Poems Are An Author's Way*.

THE PROM KING

Mitchel A. Woltersdorf, PhD, PT

Twenty years ago, freshly graduated from Northwestern University's School of Physical Therapy, my new white polyester smock with the triangular patch and I traipsed off to work at our first job in a community hospital in northwest Chicago, where we found ourselves attached to a rehabilitation service responsible for the treatment of patients with cerebrovascular accidents (CVA).

For those of you not yet breathing in the early '70s: It was a time when passive range of motion (PROM) performed by the physical therapy department staff was still an art form for all patients with CVA. It was a time when most of us thought DRG was shorthand for "drug" (we now know it really means "<u>D</u>enied <u>R</u>eimbursement is the <u>G</u>oal").

I tackled my first assignment, "PROM for all CVA patients," with vigor. I mentally rehearsed anatomy lessons as I manipulated unyielding and unnaturally resistant joints and limbs. I spoke to patients as if they were alert and responsive; many were not, but we had been taught that sometimes the unconscious mind is still capable of receiving and retaining information (proven thousands of times in undergraduate classes nationwide).

Then I confronted the matter of "productivity." A treatment of full-body PROM took a PT about 20 minutes, and I needed to have my assigned 20 patients per day done, with the remainder of the day (about an hour) relegated to paperwork. To accomplish this, I created my own system that enhanced productivity by (1) prioritizing patients by difficulty (it's still a great idea to put the most difficult tasks early in the day), (2) reviewing charts daily only on the alert patients (short-cuts are still an "uh-oh"), and (3) carrying a small Dictaphone in my pocket and recording "progress phrases" on each patient as I finished, so I wouldn't have to spend time at the end of the day attempting to recall details or waste time writing twice.

I was developing into the PROM King. I pumped out 21 or 22 patients some days. Then came the fateful day.

I started my day with the unconscious patients, because they were the most difficult. Remember, I didn't review their charts before treatment (uh-oh). I talked to them as if they were rapt with interest. As I ran on my appointed rounds, the third room had its door closed, and the lights were off. I assumed the nurse had not yet performed her daily ablutions, so I entered and began manipulating Mr. Smith's (not his real name, obviously) limbs.

The spasticity was greatly diminished, so I was glad to see him getting better. I congratulated him profusely on this. I had already finished his right side and was beginning on his left upper extremity when the nurse entered the room with a physician. I looked up just in time to see her lips form the words, "Just what are you doing?"

I replied, "Mr. Smith's range of motion." She screamed, "He's been dead for an hour." I glanced down at him and then back at her, attempting to utter something witty, but nothing came out.

I bolted past the laughing physician and wondered what I could do to make up for the lost time. I wasn't sure I could charge the patient.

It was years before I realized that that incident was the beginning of my dehumanization as I attempted to fit into the demands of the health care system. I suppose no harm occurred that day, except to the naive psyche of a neophyte PT, who only later learned that the best clinicians may not be the most productive or the most system-sensitive, they just care enough for people not to rush past them. In my case, 20 years ago, I was productive but not patient-sensitive; productivity and good care do not necessarily go hand-in-hand, as some managers would have us believe. In fact, I now realize they *cannot* go hand-in-hand, unless the PT defines productivity in terms of standards of clinical practice.

I am not proud of this incident, and I know this kind of thing doesn't happen anymore, but I think it illustrates some universal truths that are strangely current.

Reprinted from PT, ©1997; 5(5):128, with the permission of the APTA.

THE STATUS OF OCCUPATIONAL THERAPY IN CANADA

Norman L. Burnette

The story of occupational therapy in Canada prior to the war does not differ very greatly from American experiences. The historically minded will find much of interest in the records of our oldest institutions for the care of the insane. I am of the opinion that activities, which might fairly be classed as occupational therapy as we now use the term, have been a part of the regime of the hospitals of the Catholic religious orders ever since their inception in Lower Canada.

A number of local factors have made possible the continuity of the work in what is now Quebec province, chief of these being the innate artistry of the French-Canadian and the culture and temperament of the Religeuse who constitute the fine nursing staff.

In the more turbulent atmosphere of English speaking Canada it is not so easy to piece together a consecutive history.

Occupational therapy has been of sporadic growth; has flourished at times in isolated spots under energetic superintendents; has suffered serious setbacks; has been at all times incessantly harried and sniped at by indignant taxpayers and indigent politicians, and was transformed overnight by the exigencies of the war into an honored if somewhat bewildered guest at the doctors' table.

Of occupational therapy in the military hospital it is not necessary to speak. The post-war expansion has been far reaching and varied in character. Work is now being done in general hospitals, sanatoria, homes for incurables, among the home bound, in workshops for epileptics and with private patients. If I am not mistaken there has been a parallel growth in the United States.

Two other activities not included in the above are worthy of separate notice because I believe they have reached a higher stage of development in Canada than elsewhere.

First, the workshops established by the government for disabled soldiers and, second, the number of independent businesses which have been launched by men who either learned a craft while under government care or who conceived a commercial idea because they were doing some sort of handiwork.

The famous "Uncle Wiggly Toys" are a good example of this. They started as a one man idea and now represent I do not know what awe inspiring sums in capitalization and output.

The first shops were opened in Toronto early in 1920 and others followed rapidly. The industries were furniture, toys, reedwork, art metal work and art leather work. Six months observation and experimentation defined the problem. It was then seen that the shops had to be organized to provide work for four distinct groups: (a) old age cases, (b) mental defectives of the non-institutional type. It was evident that attempts to retrain either of these classes would be a waste of money as they could not meet competition in the open labor market. (c) Medical cases needing varying degrees of out-patient treatment but capable of a short day's work under hygienic conditions (heart cases, bronchitis, nephritics, arrested T.B. cases). (d) Men recovering from long periods of sickness and needing a sort of mental and moral setting up exercise before taking the plunge into the open labor market. A large number of these cases were frankly cases of neuroses.

To an American visitor the most astonishing thing would be the old age cases. Those blessed old idiots who forgot their birthdays and lied like gentlemen to get into the front line—and got there!

This class now constitutes over one-half of the men employed in the government shops and, being permanent, has become a skilled working force. The Toronto shops today practically monopolize the market for hand wrought brass and copper work in Canada and do as well most beautiful silverwork, tea, coffee, and cocoa sets, communion vessels, etc. The combined output of toys from the

Reprinted with permission from Archives of Occupational Therapy, © 1923; 2(3):179–183. Edited from the original.

various shops must represent a very respectable part of all the toys produced in the Dominion.

All of the foregoing may rightly be claimed for the credit side of occupational therapy in Canada since the war. Is there another side to the picture? I think there is. In the institutional care of the insane the progress of occupational therapy is disappointing. There have, of course, been additions to the list of hospitals engaging one or two occupational workers (one or two workers among 700 or 1000 patients!). But there have also been losses. In fact the condition is in no way different from what it was 10 years ago. Progress at one point, retrogression at another, no great movement which might be dignified by the appellation of a scientific advance in the use of occupation in the treatment of mental diseases.

We are still in the post-war period of adjustment. Demands for increased government expenditure on behalf of the asylums will be met with the justifiable plea for economy. We who believe in the value of occupational therapy claim that the exclusion of occupational therapy is not an economy. Are we fully equipped in knowledge when we make claims for the therapeutic results of our practice?

I am not particularly enthusiastic over the "Expansion." I have an uncomfortable feeling that we have run away from the hard work in the field of mental diseases to holiday in the by-paths of orthopedics and social service. These things are undoubtedly laudable, but I have a suspicion that they are also easy.

I would seriously suggest that we return again to our old love and that for a while we concentrate our efforts on some quiet, earnest, research work.

I think that occupational therapy would stand a very much better chance of attaining recognition as a scientific factor in mental hygiene if we would spend time checking our data and arriving at clear cut decisions as to what were actual facts indicated by inductive methods of search, and what were merely working hypotheses.

We make specious claims for the therapy of occupation when advocating work among the insane. There remains the task of proving this by quantitative or even qualitative measurement.

The difficulties of this field of research should not deter us from entering it. Until we do so we will never be sure of holding ground over which we have advanced because we are armed with nothing more than speculative theories.

SHOW US YOUR CREDENTIALS

Allen Mason

The establishment of the Society of Trained Masseuses in 1894 formalised "that branch of the nursing profession which has hitherto been conducted practically without status, or certificates of value to the public."

But while some felt that some form of organisation and registration was desirable, others counselled caution. Before 1894, there was no official qualification in massage. Some individuals enrolled at privately-run "schools" of massage; while others were "trained," often sketchily, by physicians—Dr Playfair at The London Hospital for example, Dr Henry Tibbits, and the aptly-named Dr Stretch Dowse among them.

But there was little chance for women, unless they had considerable hospital or private connections, to make a living solely from massage. Many of them drifted into the more profitable world of the massage parlour and prostitution.

If there was to be an official register of masseuses, then it would be impossible to exclude those with certificates signed by registered medical practitioners. This could be construed as giving approval to prostitution.

The Lancet stated that it did not wish to make moral judgements but felt, at least, that massage

Reprinted with permission from Physiotherapy, © 1992; 78(12):903. Edited from the original.

parlours and brothels should not be allowed to advertise medical treatments, when it was clear that they offered nothing of the kind.

Many journals and papers, in fact, showed a glorious disregard for any distinction there might be between medicine and prostitution. One correspondent to the *British Medical Journal* complained that he had read in the newspaper that "Madame X assisted by Nurses Y and Z receive patients daily": all, he noted, within easy reach of clubland.

The *Morning Post* was, apparently, the worst offender in this matter, but even *The Times* was not entirely innocent. An advertisement in the Agony Column in 1896 read as follows:

St Christopher's Massage Institute.
Electricity, massage, discipline and light baths.
Nurse Elizabeth at 11 St Christopher's Street, Piccadilly.

In an attempt to settle the issues, the *British Medical Journal* supplied the police with details of several massage parlours where it felt the masseuses were straying on to medical territory. The Home Secretary, however, felt that the *BMJ* was merely raising a storm in a tea-cup, and that no further action should be taken.

The massage parlour was not a Victorian invention. One historian tells us of similar facilities provided for weary Crusaders!

FEAR OF FLUNKING

Charles DiMaggio, PA-C

When the notice came in the mail, my first thought was that there must be some mistake. Six years? I looked at my certificate. Yes, 6 years. I had to take my recertification exam. Despair cast its gloomy shadow over me. One bright spot though—I didn't have to take the exam for 6 months. I mentally filed the notice under "things I'd rather not think about for a while."

But the deadline for paying the exam fee did what deadlines always do: it arrived. As I wrote the check, I realized I now had only 3 months. Despair sauntered into my life again, and this time he brought along his buddy, fear. Fear had a few things to tell me: "Do you realize that medicine is a mind-boggling body of knowledge? I bet all those texts and notes collecting dust in your study are laughably outdated. It won't be so bad losing your certification; I hear Burger King is hiring." Fear and despair assured me they had no prior commitments and would be glad to hang around until the exam.

Acclimating myself to the slings and arrows of outrageous fortune and all that, I decided to take arms against this annoying exam. My first step was to break out all those journals I had promised myself I would read someday. Six years' worth of journals is an awesome sight. Right off the bat I found an article on study techniques for the recertification exam. Now I was cooking with gas. First, the author said, begin laying out a plan about a year before the exam. It may as well have said, "First, travel back in time about 1 year." I could hear fear and despair chuckling.

The next day, I ran out and bought a review book. I was amazed after taking the first practice exam. How could I possibly know so little? Was I in some sort of suspended animation for the past 6 years, my body practicing medicine while my mind was cryogenically preserved? My friend Kev the bus driver could do better. (I made a mental note to ask Kev how difficult the bus drivers' exam was.)

I got some consolation from learning that I would not lose my certification if I didn't pass the exam. I would be "invited" to sit for the exam again in 2 years. As the rules stood, I could be "invited" to take the exam every 2 years for the rest of my life,

Reprinted from Physician Assistant, © 1992; 16(9):15, with permission of the author.

a perpetual purgatory of review tests and K-type questions. Oh death, where is thy sting?

The studying began that night and continued unabated for 3 months. I read texts, journals, and review books. I made notes. I made notes of notes and then condensed those notes onto index cards. I condensed those index cards onto smaller index cards. I thought if I kept on this way, I would eventually condense all of medicine onto one 3 × 5 index card.

An interesting thing happened. I began to enjoy the things I was learning. I was losing friends and influencing enemies with my new fund of knowledge. Most important, my differential diagnoses were clearer and more logical than they had ever been. I was able to tell patients more about their conditions.

Well, the exam came and went. I haven't received the results yet. I won't jinx myself by saying it wasn't that bad. Fear and despair left. They had appointments with a new batch of PAs. But something fundamental remained. I read my journals now. I even read texts. I look up interesting cases, just as I did when I was a student. After all, my patients deserve that much. And the years go by fast. It's never too early to start studying.

PERSONAL REFLECTIONS

Tricia Hoare, RTNM

I once worked in a nuclear medicine department whose premises lay entirely within an x-ray department and whose personnel consisted of one person—me. It was with some trepidation that I went to work on my first day—I hardly knew where to find the department within the hospital, I didn't really know any of the x-ray techs, I'd never seen the department's particular brand of nuclear medicine equipment before, and I didn't have a clue how I was going to move stretcher patients all by myself.

Much to my relief, the first person I saw that morning was the one x-ray tech with whom I had at least a bare acquaintance. She immediately showed me where the coffee pot was (in the biggest staff room I'd ever seen—it now houses a C.T. scanner) and announced that if I were going to keep arriving at work at 7:30 a.m., I had better learn where the coffee was so that I could take over her job of making the first pot of the day.

Over the next few days, I learned a number of important tasks particular to this department, such as helping one of the techs pick which tie to wear in the morning (doorknobs doubled as tie racks), staying clear of the bathroom near the barium room, and learning what a bucky is.

One afternoon at coffee, one of my colleagues said something about the bucky on the XYZ machine. I very quietly asked what a bucky was, and this seemingly innocent question was greeted with peals of laughter. When they had all stopped howling at my ignorance, I was very patiently shown a bucky, a film cassette and how a control panel worked. It wasn't long after this first lesson that I learned the significance of all the door-slamming that went on whenever I spent the morning in the darkroom. It turned out they felt that if I was going to monopolize the darkroom all morning (I couldn't use their safelight, so it seemed I was fumbling around in the dark forever), the least I could do was learn how to stamp a chest x-ray film and put it in the processor. After that, it didn't take long until my x-ray colleagues began to draw a "nosepiece" and two "arms" on my corrected and uncorrected floods, making my daily quality control images into a pair of dark glasses. They got right into inspecting my daily floods—to the point where they would even pass judgement on their quality: "Tricia, why do the nice circles look like Swiss cheese today?" was a particularly dreaded question, as was, "Tricia, why do the

Reprinted with permission of the author and Canadian Journal of Medical Radiation Technology, © 1992; 23(2):99–100.

straight line pictures have a big curve in the middle of them?"

I learned a lot from these techs, but it was also a two-way street. For their part, they learned about half-life and milking the cow. I did a reasonably good job of explaining to them that rather than shooting the radiation through a patient to expose a film, I injected the "hot stuff" (their terminology) into the patient and then detected the emitted radiations with a machine, which, via some electronic wizardry, produced those little people on the film (bone scan). At least I thought I'd explained it well, until one of them came to help me move a patient that I had just finished imaging and wanted multiple assurances that she wouldn't be exposed to any radiation (she was then in her pre-pregnant paranoia stage).

Seriously, though, there was a very special relationship in that department between x-ray and nuclear medicine—a sharing, supportive atmosphere that I wish all members could establish in their departments and hospitals.

WHY I DON'T TEACH HIGH SCHOOL CHEMISTRY

Anonymous

As my college years drew close to an end and I asked myself what career I should pursue in the years to come, I found myself troubled by a recurrent nightmare. In my dream I would make a decisive career choice. My mind full of chemistry and biology, I would return to my native Quaker Ridge and apply for a teaching job at the local high school. I would see the principal figuratively rubbing his hands with glee as he read my credentials, and he would say on the spot, "I've got just the job for you!" He would shove a contract under my nose, and say, "Sign here." The one note of pleasure in the dream was that the salary he offered was higher than I expected, and, without reading the fine print too carefully, I would promptly sign the document and rush home to my wife, singing my college song, "Oh, we have the stuff the people say."

As it does in dreams, the scene swiftly moved to the first day of school, which seemed to begin auspiciously enough, as the pupils trooped into the classroom, their faces scrubbed and shining. I would start right in, and, as I mustered my most pedagogic face, I would start to talk about how the ancient Greeks had glimmerings of the atomic nature of matter. It was then, night after night, that the nightmarish quality of the dream would assert itself. My teaching—brilliant in my own dream world—would be interrupted by a student messenger carrying a note from the principal commanding my presence.

The scene would change again, as quickly as in a movie, and I would see the principal, his face in a Cheshire Cat grin. "I hope that you read your contract carefully," he would say, "and I wonder what your plans are." I would be bewildered, but speaking in a pleasant tone, he would pretend I knew what he was talking about. "You know," he would say, "Quaker Ridge hasn't enough money to pay all the high salaries that teachers demand, but we have worked out an excellent scheme. You will, of course, apply to the State Department of Education for a research grant—say, for example, to study whether learning chemistry is influenced by the time of day that the class is held. I'd suggest that you apply for 60 percent of your salary to conduct this study. And it would be a good idea to apply for alternative support to three or four foundations. You can easily make up the rest of your salary by starting a private practice, tutoring those students

Reproduced from Journal of Laboratory and Clinical Medicine, © 1991; 117(2):87–88, with permission from Mosby, Inc.

in your classes who can't meet our high standards without a little extra help."

The nightmare would deepen. The Department of Education would tell me that it was uninterested in my grant application. Nor, in my dream, would I have any better luck with several foundations, all of which would say that I had good ideas but they needed to see preliminary results before they would even read the application. Always I would awaken with a cold sweat and a large dose of anxiety.

Well versed in the meaning of dreams from an earlier experience in bible studies, I took them for an omen. Whatever I did, I must avoid being a high school teacher, at least in a system with so bizarre a fiscal structure and so seemingly uncommitted to its function. Better to be a doctor as I knew my parents would wish. If I wanted to be a teacher, as my dreams implied, I could then pursue an academic career. I borrowed from anyone I could, applied successfully to medical school, completed three years of residency and four more years of specialized training, and happily obtained a much-coveted position at a much-coveted medical school. My chief, a pleasant and extraordinarily competent physician and investigator, called me in. "You understand," he said in his pleasantest tone, "the Medical School has no funds to support salaries for researchers, and precious little for teaching activities. I suggest that you apply to the National Institutes of Health for a research grant that might cover, say, 60 percent of your salary; alternative support can be looked for from any number of foundations. You can easily make up the rest by seeing private patients."

I wondered about a system with so bizarre a fiscal structure, and about the commitment of the Medical School to its function. And I wondered whether it was an inspired idea to become a medical school academician. As the great Yogi Berra said, it was deja vu all over again.

"THE SHOW MUST GO ON"

Cecil Birtcher

I can no longer stomach the gaudy dramas of stage, screen and story in which the plot is built around one of its own male or female celebrities, who in spite of hell, high water, 108°F temp., plain hangover, or death of dear old Daddy, still with phenomenal courage and a heart at least as large as a zeppelin, goes on with a frozen smile to do his part, dance, sing or walk a tightrope. "The Show must go on" PHOOEY! Most of them would have fared better had the audience simply been refunded its money. Certainly it would have been no world-shaking or even city-block-shaking event had the show failed to open at all. It's simply a device by which a group of diffident hams endeavor to bolster a decadent ego and by mighty chest thumpings delude the public into the spurious idea that the entertainment profession is made up of a great collection of guys and gals worthy of public panegyrics. I'm nauseated with the self-canonization of symphony conductors and tap dancers, opera prima donnas and lion tamers, dramatic dolls and trapeze artists and all of their ilk, most of whom carried on the show simply to avoid being docked come pay day.

I know many Physicians, Therapists, Nurses, Technicians and Stenographers under similar and most poignant circumstances carrying on for days, weeks, and even years in uninspired jobs. I even know a few such unglamorous characters as businessmen who doggedly keep their show going, both for a fast buck or actually for a sense of responsibility toward fellow workers. Well, look around—you are probably rubbing shoulders each day with these people who keep a show going and who expect no music, flowers, or neon lights.

Reprinted from Physical Therapy, © 1955; 35(9):472, with the permission of the APTA.

WHOSE BALLOON IS EXPANDING?

Art Labelle, DDS

Man, oh man are things expanding these days. We've got expandable trailers, expandable bras, expandable air bags in cars, and even expandable auxiliaries in dentistry.

Not too long ago we had just plain hygienists and just plain assistants and just plain technicians, but now we've got the RDH and the RDA and the CDT and the RDA (EF) and the RDH (EF) and the CDA and Lord knows what other combination of letters and numbers. What's going on here? Is it just the modern trend to expand? Is it a fascination with titles and bigger demands for salary?

For years and years and years the dental profession as a group has been guilty of the grossest kind of big bossism imaginable. Our predecessors of the last century and the early part of this century practiced what I call "solistic" dentistry, which means they did it all. They answered the phone, cast the inlays, made the appointments, and worked their magic in a sea of saliva diminished only slightly by a half-plugged saliva ejector. My father, God bless him, worked in that fashion for 42 years, and some of that ancient dentistry is still chomping away in my mouth after 40 years and more.

But we moderns need help. Gradually, over the last half century or so, we have progressed from the "solistic" approach to today's TEAM approach. We do four-handed, six-handed, eight-handed dentistry; and we hire assistants and hygienists and technicians by the bus load. We worship the great idol called PRODUCTIVITY, and we insist that we keep ourselves parked on the peak of the pyramid composed of all of these crowds in our employ.

After all, we have anointed hands.

And we are THE BOSS.

Now, much to our great chagrin, we've discovered that some of the people we've thought of as dummies have some brains and some talents. It's been shown with reliability that hygienists can be quickly taught to prepare teeth for restorations and that they can do it as well as dentists, and in some cases, better. And it's been shown that dental assistants can be rapidly taught to place and carve restorations as well as dentists. All of these preparers and carvers and fabricators are under the direct supervision of the dentist, of course, but the fact remains that objective judgment has shown that our sacrosanct talents are not exclusive.

"Holy mouth mirror," says the new young dentist. "What are you trying to do to me? Why are you training all these people, when I'm starving from lack of patients? If you keep this up, I'll have to work alone with a saliva ejector on my one patient per day while some razzmatazz character downtown employs 76 expanded staffers and sees 800 people per day."

Well, we can't have that, now can we? Dentists starving while paradental people swarm into the mouth? Let's stop all this. Let's forget the whole thing and go back to the old way. It's okay to have helpers, but let's not get carried away.

Sorry, doctor, it's too late for that. Like just about everything else in life, you can't go back to the way it was. Our helpers have begun to taste the sweetness of accomplishment, and they have been recognized by certain of us as talented people, and they have—some of them—even risen above poverty-level wages. So they aren't going to let go. And, in fact, they want more. Far too many of their numbers were stepped on for too long by too many of us, so you can't blame them for marching forward with determination to succeed and be significant.

What to do? Oh woe is me, what to do?

There are all kinds of answers, but the only one that makes any sense involves sensitivity to one's fellow man and sensitivity to one's environment. If the various members of the profession (and that includes the paradental people, too) sat down together and approached the problem intelligently, we could develop all kinds of ways to deliver our services to the public at a reasonable cost, while providing stature, accomplishment, recognition, economic reward, and a bright future for all of us.

Reprinted with permission from California Dental Association Journal, © 1978, July. Edited from the original.

We won't do it, of course, because we all have ancient prides and because it's easier to make war than make peace, where some concessions are often necessary. We could do great things just by talking to each other and forgetting the innuendo of superior-inferior relationships. But we won't, because that means having an open mind, and our minds seem to be closed. Even the omnipresent government interference is not mind opening.

Anybody got a pin for this balloon?

A HISTORY OF GREECE IN ONE PAGE

F. Clarke Fraser

Grecian culture began very B.C., in Crete and the surrounding islands, and for a while everyone got along just fine. There were no fortifications, or other signs of strife, and people just made love and pottery, not war. But the territorial instinct is strong, and as the culture spread to the mainland, the country became divided into various city states. Each had an acropolis, with a temple dedicated to one of their many gods and goddesses, all of whom seemed to be, for some reason, related to Zeus.

The excavated statues provide much useful information about these civilizations. It's no wonder that so many men got killed, the way they ran around bare naked, brandishing swords and shields, without even a jockstrap for protection down there. We saw many who had, indeed, suffered penile amputations. There were also many cases of nasal destruction, presumably due to congenital syphilis, or leprosy. And many of the statues were malformed, with no head (anencephaly) or missing arms or legs (acheiropodia). Had the Greeks developed thalidomide? They certainly seemed to have developed genetic engineering. We saw statues of women with hen's feet, referred to as harpies, and men with horse's asses, termed centaurs. Other terms, not fit to mention, were applied to men who *were* horse's asses.

Anyway, the excavations are now a major attraction for tourists, who flock to Greece from all over the world, to be reminded of how silly it is to try and get along with your neighbors by killing them.

American Journal of Medical Genetics, © 1997; 69(3):341. Reprinted by permission of Wiley-Liss, Inc., a subsidiary of John Wiley & Sons, Inc. Edited from the original.

A LOOK BACK: HISTORY OF MEDICINE

2000 BC. Here, eat this root.

1000 AD. That root is heathen. Here, say this prayer.

1850 AD. That prayer is superstition. Here, drink this potion.

1940 AD. That potion is snake oil. Here, swallow this pill.

1985 AD. That pill is ineffective. Here, take this antibiotic.

2000 AD. That antibiotic does not work any more. Here, eat this root. (Author unknown.)

Reprinted with permission from Journal of Emergency Nursing, © 1999; 25(2):157.

WORD PLAY

Probably the first joke you ever learned to tell was some variation of a play on words. Since you've become a sophisticated health care professional, that simple joy of using language is now limited to a particular profession and more likely to be written than verbal. Let's hope that your tastes have matured and you're not still telling colleagues knock-knock jokes. No matter how seasoned we may appear though, there still remains plenty of room in our jargon-filled lives for the simple pleasure of playing with language and for a sharp turn of phrase.

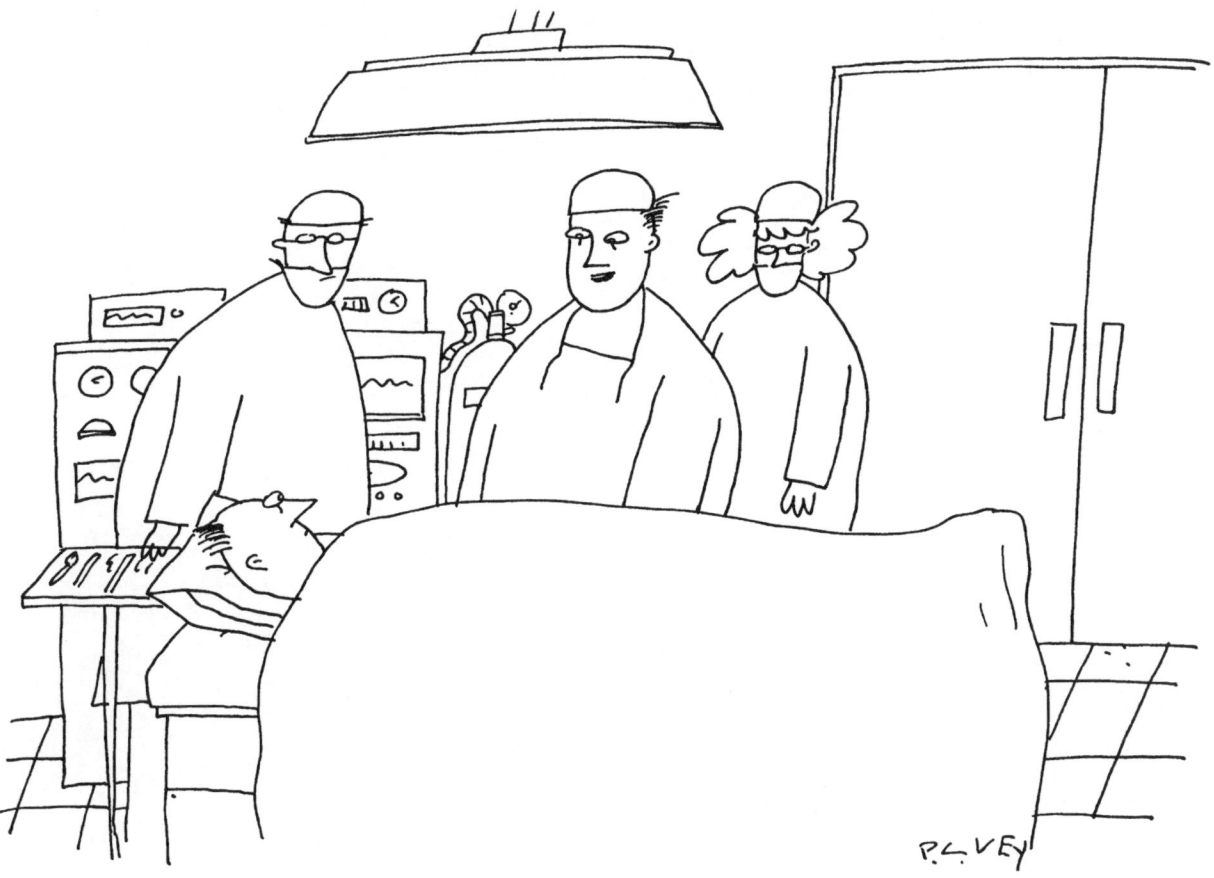

"I've decided to play God today, I hope you don't mind."

© 2000 P.C. Vey from cartoonbank.com. All Rights Reserved.

ACRONYMITIS, ANACHRONIPHOBIA, AND EUPHEMISMUS

David Wolman, PA-C

When I was a kid acronyms were shortcuts to saying Federal Bureau of Investigation or Union of Soviet Socialist Republics without having to, uh, say all that. Later, some of my college friends became familiar with one of the most famous acronyms of our generation: LSD. As a result, I have always been wary of abbreviations. To me, they have become synonymous with: You may not know what's in your Kool-Aid.

So I wasn't surprised some years ago when I began PA training to find myself swamped with acronyms, from Abd to Z—well, I can't think of one starting with Z but I'm sure there is one. Even our own profession has created a myriad of nyms: AAPA, APAP, NCCPA, SAAAPA, SEMPA. Subsequently, I've identified the syndrome: Acronymitis™.

I also quickly learned that, conversely, medical folks like to use multisyllabic words as well, usually ancient Latin and Greek, to describe simple things. I soon discovered that the medical language was one in which there was an incomprehensible mix of short telegrammatic acronyms and long, ancient, intimidating anachronisms. I refer to the latter as Anachroniphobia™.

As the years have gone by, I have noticed a proliferation of acronyms. Meanwhile, long ancient words (LAWs when acronymized) are still used when a practitioner a) wants to humiliate a student, b) is bored with acronyms, or c) has just taken some boards.

The business of medicine, simultaneously, has given us some great new acronyms (but no LAWs), such as HMO, PPO, MCO, PCO, and countless other Os to accompany your Cheerios. In a way, the history of medicine can be divided into two eras: BMCO and AMCO, standing for before MCOs and after MCOs, respectively. Perhaps the most important acronym of MCOs is DRGs. Hospitals are now using the technique of "upcoding" with DRGs to increase billings. Thus, it would appear, that acronyms and fraud are loosely connected. It is easier to cheat in code than in flowing language. We have developed a shorthand, high-tech system of virtual dishonesty.

As far as LAWs go, I think people sometimes forget that these words were invented 2000 years ago—we're not talking cutting edge, folks. There is an irony here in that modern medicine prides itself on being so up-to-date that if you walk away from your Netscape Navigator for 5 minutes the information on the screen may have changed by the time you return. So, to me, it isn't such a crime to say "red" instead of "erythematous," but erythematous makes you sound smarter.

I must admit I have rebelled against acronyms and LAWs. Recently, at work in the ED one late night, after numerous calls to PCPs, HMOs, and MRIIIs, I could not find anyone willing to take care of my patient—he had been abridged out of existence. (I think we all missed the point of President Clinton's campaign slogan: what he was really saying was "abridge" to the twenty-first century.)

I decided to try an experiment. I actually consulted the on-call orthopod (orthopod = ancient Greek word meaning training of children) attending (from the Latin meaning ornery omniscient deity) and deliberately taunted the unwary, sleepy physician (ancient Greek word *physikos*) by using simple language.

I said: "I have a good man with a bad knee."

Now this really sent the somnolent wizard into a tizzy.

"A bad knee? What part of the knee?" he bellowed into the phone.

"The patient hurts," I responded.

"What did you say?" the attending asked.

Used with permission from Physician Assistant, © 1997; 21(6):162, 164–165, Springhouse Corporation/www.springnet.com. Edited from the original.

"I said *the patient hurts*."

"Hurts?" The unwitting subject of my experiment squawked incredulously as if he had just encountered the rare idiom of a foreign language. He was confused. But not confused enough to then ask me: "Is this a ward patient? Because you can call my resident."

Ward patient? That's a euphemism, I thought to myself. In addition to acronyms and LAWs, we also have our own secret language. Ward patient is a euphemism for a patient who has no insurance, thus, if unable to dump the patient onto his resident, the on-call physician is forced to work for the sheer altruism of helping someone in need (sans DRG code), a concept that went out with the Hippocratic Oath (460? 377? BC)—about the same time acronyms and LAWs and euphemisms came in. The Hippocratic Oath was replaced by the Hypocritic Oath, which is now the accepted standard. Thus, I invented the disorder of Euphemismus™.

I then explained to the orthopod in simple terms that my patient had a fx s/p fall while ice skating with grandson c a PMH of IDDM, HTN, CAD, and a PSH of CABG×4, SH 30 pk yrs, FH colon CA with ROS neg. The radiograph demonstrated a nondisplaced, linear, horizontal fracture of the entire aspect of the intercondylar eminence. Physical exam revealed a positive Lochman's, an effusion, decreased ROM, with the distal extremity sensory and vascularly intact. The fact that my patient had been recently laid off his job of 30 years for reasons of cost cutting by a new boss fondly referred to as "Chainsaw Charlie" and dropped from the insurance pool was a piece of information I did not convey because it was irrelevant to his need for care.

"You," I further explained, meaning the orthopod, "are ON CALL. This means that, even though the patient has no insurance, in plain English, *you need to jump into your BMW and come in and practice your ancient art of healing* ASAP. You can bring your acronyms and euphemisms and your big words if you want. There'll be a forklift waiting at the door."

"And, by the way, bring some empathy, too, if your supply isn't depleted," I added.

The specialist was nonplussed. He asked me what gave me the right to speak to him in this abrupt way.

I rattled the X-ray of my patient's knee into the mouthpiece of the phone making the sound of stage thunder. I took a long, loud slurp of my stale soda, and finally answered:

"Well, sometimes a PA just *has* to assist an MD."

SOUNDINGS

Premedical Science
George Dunea

This information came over the Internet some years ago. It purports to be the answers given by students in science exams around the world. It came with the comment that "it is truly astonishing what weird science our young scholars can create under the pressure of time and grades." I was unable to trace the author, but as the work deserves wider dissemination, I present here the answers of most interest to a medical audience.

- General: "The body consists of three parts—the brainium, the borax, and the abominable cavity. The brainium contains the brain; the borax, the heart and lungs; and the abominable cavity, the bowls, of which there are five—a, e, i, o, and u."
- Respiration: "When you breathe, you inspire. When you do not breathe, you expire." "Respiration consists of two acts: first inspiration, then expectoration."

Reprinted from BMJ, © 1999; 318(7191):1153, with permission from the BMJ Publishing Group.

- Cardiovascular: "The three kinds of blood vessels are arteries, veins, and caterpillars."
- Gastrointestinal: "The alimentary canal is located in the northern part of Alabama."
- Dentistry: "A permanent set of teeth consists of eight canines, eight cuspids, two molars, and eight cuspidors."
- Orthopaedics: "The skeleton is what is left after the insides have been taken out and the outsides have been taken off. The purpose of the skeleton is something to hitch meat on."
- Reproductive medicine: "Artificial insemination is when the farmer does it to the cow instead of the bull." "To prevent contraception, wear a condominium." "Many women believe that an alcoholic binge will have no effects on the unborn fetus, but that is a large misconception."
- Haematology: "Before giving a blood transfusion, find out if the blood is affirmative or negative."
- Eyes and nose: "To remove dust from the eye: pull the eye down over the nose." "For nosebleeds, put the nose lower than the body until the heart stops." "For a cold: use an agoniser to spray the nose until it drops in your throat."
- First aid: "For fainting: rub the person's chest or, if a lady, rub her arm above the head instead. Or put the head between the knees of the nearest doctor." "For asphyxiation: apply artificial respiration until the patient is dead." "For drowning: climb on top of the person and move up and down to make artificial perspiration." "For dog bite: put the dog away for several days. If he has not recovered, then kill it."

THE DOCTOR'S DICTIONARY

Howard J. Bennett, MD

Ambrose Bierce was an American writer and satirist who was known for his incisive wit. In 1911, Bierce published *The Devil's Dictionary*, a compendium of clever, sometimes scathing definitions that commented on his times. Although his dictionary primarily consists of nonmedical words, Bierce tossed a few barbs at the medical profession:

Diaphragm *n*. A muscular partition separating disorders of the chest from disorders of the bowels.

Disease *n*. Nature's endowment to medical schools.

After spending a weekend going through Bierce's dictionary, I thought I would coin some alternative definitions of my own.

acute *adj*. Sudden, without warning. As in the pain one gets when approached by a drug rep at the end of a busy day.

aphorism *n*. An adage or wise saying, as in, "Half a nurse is better than none," or "A gallbladder in the hand is worth 2 on the floor."

atrophy *v*. To become smaller with disuse. As in the state of mind brought on by successfully matching in the residency of one's choice.

circumcision *n*. Elective surgical procedure that has continued into modern times so adolescent males can shower at school in peace.

clinical practice guidelines *n*. *Cliff's Notes* for doctors.

deferred *v*. Refers to part of the physical exam that was not done on admission. It is not likely to be done after admission either.

drug *n*. A substance that when given to a patient produces the side effect you forgot to mention.

fetal monitor *n*. Electronic device that allows obstetricians to avoid bodily fluids for as long as possible.

fever *n*. A change in body temperature that decreases a doctor's sleep but increases his income.

Reproduced with permission from *The Journal of Family Practice*, © 1999; 48(4):313.

foreign body *n.* Any object smaller than a toaster that is left in the vicinity of a young child for less than 2 minutes.

heart *n.* (orthopedic definition) A muscular organ that has the sole purpose of pumping antibiotics to the bones.

hemorrhoids *n.* The body's revenge for a high-fat diet.

informed consent *n.* The only thing that stands between a surgeon and his 9-iron.

nonpaying patients *n.* Relatives.

not really *n phr.* Expression used to dodge questions on rounds (usually when a resident forgot to do something). *Attending:* Was the patient anemic? *Resident:* Not really.

oriented x three *adj phr.* Less confused than your physician.

penis *n.* See vagina.

pimping *v.* A popular form of entertainment in medical centers, occasionally interrupted by teaching.

push, push, push *v phr.* What obstetrics nurses tell women in labor to do right before those women strangle their husbands.

rectal *n.* Part of the physical exam that illustrates the true meaning of the Yuletide maxim, "It is better to give than to receive."

scut *n.* Chores that have hypertrophied.

tenure *n.* Status granted by a medical center that guarantees employment until death or until the center is purchased by a for-profit hospital chain, whichever comes first.

unethical researcher *n.* Anyone who gets more grants than you do.

vagina *n.* Aren't you a little old to be looking up words like this?

THE VENEREAL GAME

Francis V. Hanavan

One of the curses of a misspent youth, which haunts me as I make my way through the forest of allied health, has been a near fatal exposure to a liberal arts education. To this very day, I am plagued by a fascination with words.

The venereal game is played with words (not what you expected, eh?). Today's game involves inventing terms of venery. You are of course already familiar with venery in such collective phrases that range from common expressions like a litter of puppies or swarm of bees through the more fanciful bevy of beauties or gaggle of geese or, one of my own personal favorites, a flourish of trumpets. Well, one day I got to thinking about how to play the venereal game with the allied health professions and came up with some of the following:

    A stat of medical technologists
    A series of x-ray technicians
    A file of medical records administrators
    A breath of respiratory therapists
    A flex of physical therapists
    A floss of dental hygienists
    A helping of physician's assistants
    An entrenchment of tenured faculty
    An adjustment of occupational therapists
    A clamber of assistant deans
    A twadle of deans

There, then, the gauntlet is down. Can you think of anything in your field?

Reprinted with permission from Journal of Allied Health, © 1981; 10(3):215. Edited from the original.

NEED A CHUCKLE?

Check Out These Codes

Erno S. Daniel, MD

When Medicare mandated that we use ICD-9-CM coding down to the fifth digit for everything we do, I thought I was in for dullsville, a drag, a hassle. Instead, when I sat down with the book one rainy California weekend, a whole new world of diseases opened up to me.

I had more fun that weekend than I can remember since I ran the dandy fever clinic in my residency days. Back then, we often had to enlist the chief of medicine to convince patients that dandy fever (code 061) was a real diagnosis, not a prank by the senior residents.

I was just a few pages into the thousand-page volume (not much of a plot) when I learned that adolescence and puberty (both V21.1) are internationally recognized pathologies. I was much relieved to find out that teenagers act the way they do because they're sick. Maybe it's because they spend so much time listening to that rock group, Virulent Bubo (099.0).

Most of us would agree that the adolescent proclivity for junk food is sick, so let's be grateful that we can assign the correct diagnosis of depraved appetite or starch eating (both 307.52). Maybe we'll also find a cure for such teen maladies as cluttering (307.0), yawning (786.09), and variations in hair color (704.3).

My grade-schooler and her friends have their own set of medical woes. Some suffer from spoiled child reaction or temper tantrums (both 312.1). Medical intervention may be needed to treat their timidity (313.21) on the one hand, or bullying (312.0) on the other. Cruelty in children (312.9) is a disease—a rampant one, as I recall.

At the other end of the spectrum, I was shocked to discover the incredible political incorrectness of ICD-9. Imagine that old age (797) is coded as a disease! Its alternate designation as senile debility is positively slanderous.

As the rain beat on the roof, I was pleasantly surprised to learn that I could code the whole weekend as a clouded state (780.09). Unfortunately, my wife went out for a walk and got wet feet (also known as immersion foot, or trench foot (991.4)), and a pair of shoes one of the kids left outside ended up with worm-eaten soles (102.3). We even had an invasion of red bugs (133.8) in the house. Luckily, I had a ready-made ICD-9 code to give to the exterminator.

Our whole family was a bit under the weather. My wife had a five-day fever (083.1), I had a three-day fever (066.0), and our youngest, a seven-day fever (061). Our other three children had two-day, four-day, and six-day fevers, but since these lacked ICD-9 codes, insurance wouldn't cover them. It was the beginning of winter, so we couldn't classify the ailment as spring fever (309.23).

All the codes were still fresh in my mind when I returned to the office the following Monday. Sure enough, the first patient I saw had winter vomiting disease (078.82). Good thing it was December; there's no code for summer vomiting disease. But I made a mistake and diagnosed it as Arizona enteritis (008.1), forgetting that Medi-Cal would not authorize treatment for an out-of-state problem. I should have just used the generic code for California disease (114.0).

When the pastor came in with a sore throat, I was overjoyed to find that it could be properly coded as clergyman's sore throat (784.49). But I couldn't do the same for the officer on the beat with the same symptoms; the closest I could come was policeman's disease (729.2). I was able to correctly code Davidson's anemia (284.9) for Mr. Davidson but, alas, couldn't give equal billing to Mrs. Geschnorbowitz's anemia. Meanwhile, a patient with a bald tongue (529.4) wanted to try Rogaine or Propecia.

Many of my specialist friends have managed to simplify matters. To some rheumatologists, everything is a creaking joint (719.60). A neurologist I

Copyright © 1999 by Medical Economics. Reprinted by permission from Medical Economics Magazine; 76(7):265–266.

know concludes that everyone is having either spells (780.3) or trembles (988.8). To the pulmonologist who runs the emphysema clinic, everything is a barrel chest (738.3). Speaking of specialists, the annual announcement of new salaries for our medical staff prompts the predictable epidemic of compensation neurosis (300.11).

Oh, the things you learn when you spend a few minutes with the ICD-9! It's a crime to carry a concealed weapon, but carrying a concealed penis (752.65) is a codable condition. Clumsiness (781.3) is an affliction that may qualify us for disability. If you'd had a forgettable travel experience, you can be properly diagnosed as having a bad trip (305.6).

I tried to think of a way my discoveries on that rainy day could benefit colleagues. I stayed up several nights in an attempt to distill this information into a few vital codes that could be printed on a wallet card. After much editing, I finally came up with:

Sick—799.9
Worried well—V65.5

You'll agree, I'm sure, that these codes cover any patient or medical circumstance you may encounter.

In thumbing through ICD-9 one last time, however, I was surprised to find that death is a disease. Is it considered terminal, I wondered—or manageable, reversible, or curable? Instantaneous death (798.1) is listed, but not slow death.

The latter may be what you experienced as you read this piece. Or maybe you've just had a healthy dose of corn (700).

FIFTY WAYS TO LOVE YOUR LIVER

(With Apologies to Paul Simon)
Jeffrey B. Moran

This organ's not inside your head,
she said to me.
It's in the abdomen, anatomically.
I'd like to help you understand hepatically,
There must be fifty ways to love your liver.

She said, it's really not where food
that has been chewed
Is digested into tiny molecules.
But it makes bile which into the gut is spewed.
There must be fifty ways to love your liver.

Chorus:
You just lay off the smack, Jack.
Eat some more bran, Stan.
Make the right choice, Royce,
Just listen to me.

Cut out the brew, Sue.
Don't want to be yellow, fellow.
Eat your protein, Gene,
And let your liver be.

She said, hepatitis pains your liver so,
It usually comes from viruses, you know,
In contaminated food and used hypos.
There must be fifty ways to love your liver.

She said, remember how cirrhosis
makes you bawl.
It comes from drinking too much alcohol.
And I realized that though she had a lot of gall,
There must be fifty ways to love your liver.

Chorus: as before

Reprinted with permission from Annals of Improbable Research, 1995; 1(4).

USER-FRIENDLY MICROBIOLOGICAL NOMENCLATURE

Edward M. Thompson, MD
Allen F. Shaughnessy, PharmD

In the age of digital beepers, laparoscopic surgery, and cephalosporins for everything, isn't it time we brought oil-immersion nomenclature into the 1990s?

Really, now. Do you honestly know what TWAR stands for? Can you spell the Lyme disease spirochete's name correctly? Does anyone care if you can? Has this kind of knowledge enthralled your neighbors at dinner parties?

We propose new user-friendly nomenclature; bug names that sizzle with relevance instead of obscure surnames. Looking at some recognizable but arcane names, we offer substitutes that should roll smoothly off the tongue (even if that tongue is attached to a medical student).

1. Old Name: *Borrelia burgdorferi*
   New Name: *Willie's Bug*
   Rationale: Name it for the guy's first name, for crying out loud.

2. Old Name: *Mycoplasma pneumoniae*
   New Name: *Atypicillus*
   Rationale: Easier than trying to remember whether pneumoniae ends in -a or -ae (and whether to pronounce it with a short "a," a long "a," or long "e."

3. Old Name: *Branhamella, Neisseria,* or *Moraxella catarrhalis*
   New Name: *Makeupyermindalis*
   Rationale: This will allow for future transmogrification of this wily critter.

4. Old Name: TWAR
   New Name: TWERP
   Rationale: **T**he **W**atchamacallit **E**tiology for **R**esearch **P**neumonia.

5. Old Name: *Bacteroides fragilis* (aka *B frag*)
   New Name: *B hardy*
   Rationale: It's not "fragilis" against most antibiotics.

6. Old Name: Methicillin-resistant *Staphylococcus aureus*
   New Name: *Staphylococcus turfalis*
   Rationale: A "turf" to the infectious disease service is what we want to do with this anyway.

7. Old Name: *Chlamydia trachomatis*
   New Name: *Q-tipicus*
   Rationale: The patient's eyes are already big when he sees it.

8. Old Name: *Escherichia coli*
   New Name: *Good n' Plentycus*
   Rationale: Reminds us what they look like.

9. Old Name: *Gonococcus*
   New Name: *Claptocockus*
   Rationale: Let's put it in terms our patients can understand.

10. Old Name: *Staphylococcus saprophiticus*
    New Name: *Sowhaticus*
    Rationale: We see it on cultures, but no one knows what to do with it.

11. Old Name: *Pseudomonas aeruginosa*
    New Name: *Stinkyonas*
    Rationale: It's the initiation smell for interns.

12. Old Name: *Salmonella typhi*
    New Name: *Squirtsinella*
    Rationale: They look nothing like salmon.

13. Old Name: Hepatitis A, Hepatitis B, Hepatitis C, Hepatitis D, Hepatitis non-W non-X, etc
    New Name: Hepatitis Ann, Hepatitis Bill, Hepatitis Cindy, Hepatitis Don, etc
    Rationale: They already do it for hurricanes.

14. Old Name: *Yersinia pestis*
    New Name: *Yersinia pestis*
    Rationale: Some names are just too good to change.

15. Old Name: _____ (etiological agent for Alzheimer's disease)
    New Name: _____
    Rationale: We'll forget it anyway.

Reproduced with permission from *The Journal of Family Practice*, © 1998; 46(1):89.

PROFESSIONALISM AND SONO "TECHS"

Linda M. Chase, BA, BS, RDMS

Sonographers have long been concerned about the way they are perceived by the medical community. Over the years, we have achieved not only professional status, but respect and approbation from other medical professionals. This is good. However, there is still one aspect of sonography that does not appear to be consistent with this general trend. That is the use of the term "tech" to denote the professional sonographer or echocardiographer.

Although much effort has been made to encourage both the medical community and the general public to use the terms "sonographer" and "echocardiographer," it seems to be a losing battle, since sonographers and echocardiographers still refer to themselves as "techs." To find a solution to this problem, I think we must first look at why this is happening. Could it be that these professional sonographers really think of themselves as "techs?" Do they regard their role as merely that of a picture-taker, a minor functionary in the otherwise elevated realm of diagnosis? Does not being "one of the boys (read 'techs')" make them uncomfortable? I think not. Certainly, the sonographers I know seem to think very highly of themselves. So what is the difficulty?

What we need is some kind of short, pithy term which will satisfy both professional and practical requirements. Once such a word is found, it should catch on in no time. The problem is finding the best term to use. Actually, it is not a real problem, since, as speakers of American English, we have several tried and true options open to us. We can borrow words from other languages, we can use acronyms, or we can invent any word we choose to call ourselves.

As far as the first option goes, we have already used both Greek and Latin to form the words "sonographer" and "echocardiographer," and the other languages from which English has traditionally borrowed, such as Spanish, French, and German, all tend to use lengthy descriptive phrases. Imagine trying to fit Ultraschallbehandschriftenkunder into one of the aforementioned sentences. However, there is at least one refreshing alternative. We have to look no further than our forebears for the Old English term "swogwrāt," which means literally "noise writer," for a terrific, short, pithy term, one which would be sure to catch on.

Our second choice, the use of an acronym, is inordinately American and would thus provide us not only with a new and different title, but would highlight our patriotism. Not only that, but the very act of inventing the best acronym could provide hours of entertainment, while waiting for patients to arrive, for example, and could lead to contests compared with which the Lottery would seem a mere trifle. The following are some acronym suggestions.

Acronyms may serve merely to define:
PRUNE Professional Registered Ultrasonographer and Noninvasive Echocardiographer
RUMP   Registered Ultrasound Medical Professional
PRUDE Professional Registered Ultrasonographer and Diagnostic Echocardiographer

Acronyms may indicate level of performance:
The Student
PEST   Professional Echocardiographer and Sonography Trainee
The Tyro
CUB   Capable Ultrasound Beginner

Acronyms may indicate other levels of proficiency:
JESTER Journeyman Echocardiography and Sonography Trainee
SOSO   Sonographic Operator—Somewhat Optimal
MESS   Master Echocardiographic and Sonographic Specialist
TOUT   Transcendentally Outstanding Ultrasound Technologist

Even Job descriptions:
CHUMP Capable Head Ultrasound Managerial Professional

Reprinted with permission from Journal of Diagnostic Medical Sonography, © 1991; 7(6):321–322. Edited from the original.

Our last option, that of actually making up whatever term we wish to be called, gives us the most latitude, but presents some problems. What are our parameters? (We ultrasound professionals are always concerned with parameters.) Do we limit ourselves to words that are ultrasound related? Or, in the spirit of freedom and democracy and the American way of life, do we allow ourselves the latitude to make up anything we want? In other words, do we admit artistic license into the hallowed world of science? A heady question, and one that is not to be treated lightly. Or, should I say, one that must be treated soundly?

Of course, there are always those who really don't care what you call them, as long as you call them to dinner. Well, soup's on, you swogwrāts.

RIDICULITIS: MORE [SIC] HUMOR

John H. Dirckx, MD

TABLE 1. *Responses to questions on a medical history sheet*

Any known allergies to food or medicines	Surgical Operations (cont.)
Allergic to non-allergenic stitches	Warts removed, not very important
Horse syrum	Serious illness or injury requiring hospitalization
Known	or prolonged treatment
Ruffage (to much)	Asthma—cured
Current medicines	Back disc Lombardi
Antibodities	Bilateral reflexes of the ureters
Anthropine	Brown out, low sugar
Deflammatories	Coronation of the aortia
Dialating drops	Focal glomergular neuphritis
Ibruphrophan	Exherted asthma
Pregnizone	Have infrequent fainting spells for life
Quartisone	Implanted moller
Sutafederine (pseudoephedrine)	I have football headaches. If I get hit in the head
Surgical Operations	I have a migrain headache which could lead
A bumb was taken off the inside of my lip	to a concussion or even coma.
Auxilliary nervicular bone in foot	I tore all 3 ligaments in my knee
Brocken leg, tonsoils, endometreous	Kidney disorter (nephritis)
Had appendix removed, but not for appendicitis	Left hand metacarple fell on
I have had my appendicitis removed	Leg—stressed fracture
Left knee—stitches—weak bones underneath	Mesenteric adontitis
Malrotation of the bowls	Microplasmal pneumonia
Mental plate in rt arm	My chin/ankle area bothering me
Plastic surgery to reattach nose	Nose shattered
Removal of back wisdom teeth	Polycystitis
Removal of indescendant left testicle at birth	Scar tissue on left temporal area causing
Right handle middle forefinger	numbness of left side
Testical drop	Scarlet tina
Tumor in right humorous	Slight appendicitis
200 stitches received from running through a	Tempra Mandibular Jaw (TMJ)
sliding glass door	Test for sugar in urine; slightly high
Velacose seal removed	Thought distortion

Reprinted with permission from American Journal of Dermatopathology, © 1998; 20(4):425–427. Edited from the original.

CHARTING CHUCKLES

Jan Black, RN, OCN

At one time or another, every health care professional has probably charted a note or two that didn't come out quite right. These bloopers were collected from medical records across the country.

Cardiac

- Patient has chest pains if she lies on her left side for over a year.
- By the time she was admitted to the hospital, her rapid heart had stopped and she was feeling much better.

Musculoskeletal

- On the second day, the knee was better, and on the third day, it had completely disappeared.
- While in the emergency department, she was examined, X-rated, and sent home.

Neurologic

- Patient was alert and unresponsive.
- Healthy appearing, decrepit 69-year-old female, mentally alert, but forgetful.
- She is numb from her toes down.
- When she fainted, her eyes rolled around the room.

Gastrointestinal

- Rectal examination revealed a normal-sized thyroid.
- The patient had waffles for breakfast and anorexia for lunch.
- She stated that she had been constipated for most of her life until 1989, when she got a divorce.
- Bleeding started in the rectal area and continued all the way to Los Angeles.
- The patient was to have a bowel resection. However, he took a job as a stockbroker instead.
- Fleet enema given with stool hard as pine knots.
- Patient complains of indigestion since last night when he ate a stake.
- Patient passed flatus . . . two short, one long.
- Patient was seen in consultation by the physician, who felt we should sit tight on the abdomen, and I agreed.

Gynecologic/Urologic

- Examination of genitalia reveals that he is circussized.
- Indwelling urinary catheter draining clear yellow roses.
- Examination of genitalia was completely negative except for the right foot.
- Pelvic examination to be done later on the floor.
- Indwelling urinary catheter draining large amount of urine the color of American beer.
- MD at bedside attempting to urinate. Unsuccessful. (The physician was actually attempting to intubate.)

Social History

- The patient lives at home with his mother, father, and pet turtle, who is presently enrolled in day care three times a week.
- Patient was in his usual state of good health until his airplane ran out of gas and crashed.
- Examination reveals a well-developed male lying in bed with his family in no distress.

Miscellaneous

- The skin was moist and dry.
- Both breasts are equal and reactive to light and accommodation.

Used with permission from Black, J., Nursing 97; 27(12):53, © Springhouse Corporation/www.springnet.com.

- The baby was delivered; the cord clamped and cut and handed to the pediatrician, who breathed and cried immediately.
- Skin: somewhat pale, but present.
- I saw your patient today, who is still under our car for physical therapy.
- Because she can't get pregnant with her husband, I thought you'd like to work her up.
- The test indicated abnormal lover function.
- If he squeezes the back of his neck for 4 or 5 years, it comes and goes.
- Discharge status: alive, but without permission.

MORE CHARTING CHUCKLES

Jan Black, RN, OCN

How's That Again?

- Occasional, constant, infrequent headaches.
- The patient left the hospital feeling much better, except for her original complaints.
- The patient is tearful and crying constantly. She also seems depressed.
- Patient has left his white blood cells at another hospital.
- She slipped on the ice and apparently her legs went in separate directions last December.
- Patient was released to outpatient department without dressing.
- Patient expired on the floor uneventfully.
- The left leg became numb at times and she walked it off.
- Patient lying on left side in no apparent distress with no complaints watching *Soul Train*.
- Diagnosis: uninhabited neurogenic bladder.

Patient/Physician Relationships

- The patient has been depressed ever since she began seeing me in 1983.
- I'll be happy to go into her gastrointestinal system; she seems ready and anxious.
- The patient will need disposition, and therefore, we will get Dr. Blank to dispose of him.
- Patient was admitted through the emergency department. I examined her on the floor.
- Between you and me, we ought to be able to get this lady pregnant.

History Lessons

- The patient has no past history of suicides.
- The patient's past medical history has been remarkably insignificant with only a 40-pound weight gain in the past 3 days.
- Coming from Detroit, this man has no children.

The Lovin' Feeling

- The patient had had no rigors or shaking chills, but her husband states she was very hot in bed last night.
- The patient experienced sudden onset of severe shortness of breath with a picture of acute pulmonary edema at home while having sex, which gradually deteriorated in the emergency department.

Just Follow the Directions

- I've suggested to the patient that he loosen his pants before standing and then, when he stands with the help of his wife, they should fall to the floor.

Patients Say the Darndest Things

- Patient states there is a burning pain in his penis, which goes to his feet.
- Patient refused an autopsy.
- "Doc! Is it broke or just fractured?"

Used with permission from Black, J., Nursing 98; 28(5):64, © Springhouse Corporation/www.springnet.com.

Word Play

A Funny Thing Happened on the Way to the ED

Medical professionals aren't the only people who make the occasional misstatement. The following remarks were written on insurance forms by people involved in automobile accidents:

- The guy was all over the road. I had to swerve a number of times before I hit him.
- I pulled away from the side of the road, glanced at my mother-in-law, and headed for the embankment.
- An invisible car came out of nowhere, struck my vehicle, and vanished.
- In an attempt to hit a fly, I drove into a telephone pole.
- I was thrown from the car as it left the road. I was later found in a ditch by some stray cows.
- The indirect cause of this accident was a little guy in a small car with a big mouth.

"RAAT"

The Rehabilitation Acronym and Abbreviation Test

John Dolan, RhD
Ralph E. Matkin, RhD

The Test

Rehabilitation Acronym and Abbreviation Test (RAAT)

Abbreviated Form

CORE represents which organization?
a) Commission of Rehabilitation Experts
b) Commission on Rehabilitation Education
c) Council on Radio and Electronics

A document used in education which is similar to the IWRP in rehabilitation.
a) Note From Home (NFH)
b) Report Card (RC)
c) Individualized Education Plan (IEP)

Two organizations representing private rehabilitation practitioners
a) RSA and JARC
b) CARF and JCAH
c) NARPPS and CARP

The real organization using the abbreviation "WFD"
a) World Federation of the Deaf
b) Western Football Division
c) Women's Federation for the Disabled

SEARS is to DOE as NAIL is to...
a) SSA
b) NRA
c) HAMMER

Select the answer that is one of the railroads in the game "Monopoly"
a) A&TBCB
b) MDTA
c) B&O

Depending on whom you address, DOT can represent either the Department of Transportation or...
a) Dictionary of Occupational Titles
b) Difficult or Time-consuming
c) Don't Offend Tyrants

Reprinted with permission from Journal of Rehabilitation, © 1983; 49(1):75–77. Edited from the original.

AFB represents . . .
a) Affectionate Fuzzy Bunny
b) Air Force Base
c) American Foundation for the Blind

RCB is to ARCA as . . .
a) ALAN is to ALDA
b) JARC is to NRCA
c) HEATH is to CANDY

AGDIR is not listed but represents . . .
a) Another Great Day in Rehabilitation
b) All Good Drinkers Imbibe Religiously
c) A Gosh-Darned Insensitive Rehabilitationist

Answers
1. b
2. c
3. c
4. a
5. b
6. c
7. a
8. c
9. b
10. a

AN EDUCATOR CALLS FOR A STANDARDIZATION OF TERMS:

Taking the Fat Out of Respiratory Care's Alphabet Soup

Joseph G. Sorbello MEd, RRT

As respiratory care practitioners, we all know the "alphabet soup" that exists for health care in general and respiratory care in particular. As I was teaching one of our program's spring courses "Prolonged Artificial Ventilation" and during our summer ventilator laboratories, it struck me once again how confusing the terms, acronyms, and abbreviations can be—confusing to the point of being ridiculous. Even well-defined and complete explanations in professionally prepared material can be confusing and, perhaps, amusing—particularly to the person with little background in the field's jargon. To illustrate, I compiled the following.

Airway Pressure Therapy & Alphabet Soup

First came IPPB, CPPB, C, A/C, ZEEP, NEEP, PEEP, and sPEEP. Then IMV, SIMV, CPAP, NPPV, HFPPV, HFJV, HFO, IPV, VDR, and HBO. Eventually we got to CMV, AMV, EMMV, MMV, PSV, PCV, PCIRV, APRV, CDAP, PRVC, VS, ECMO, IVOX, and TGI. Coming at us is PAV, PLV, FLV, and NO.

RCPs and MDs are familiar with both PVS and FVS, which are forms of MAV. Now comes BiPAP™ S/T-D with APM and DCP where you may observe OFL on the LED. You may use S, ST, or T using BiPAP, CPAP, IPAP, or EPAP. The LED on the DCP will display BPM, OFL, and TV.

When using T, you must adjust % IPAP time for an acceptable I:E, IPAP, EPAP, and BPM, but make sure you turn on the APM first. When initiating or weaning you may increase or decrease IPAP and/or EPAP by 2 centimeters at a time. In emergencies you must do all of the above ASAP to augment FRC in order to raise S_{aO_2} and P_{aO_2} while lowering P_{aCO_2}, thereby stabilizing pH. Monitoring of HR, BP, RR, and EKG is also recommended. Perhaps all of this will culminate in a lowering of the WOB_I, as seen on the P/V loop.

All of this can be reviewed by looking at a VHS from the AARC on VCRs attached to TVs. Maybe someday soon someone will put all of this on CD-ROM and incorporate it into CAI and VR!

Remember that BiPAP™ S/T-D may also be used PRN, OK?

Reprinted with permission from Respiratory Care, © 1994; 39(7): 772–773. Edited from the original.

WE'RE ALL IN THIS TOGETHER

At some point, almost everyone wonders what it would have been like had they chosen another professional field. Looking from the outside, some of our colleagues' work days seem so idyllic, peaceful, and calm. If only our own career paths could occasionally lead to some of those same qualities. However, even if you were to change careers, the faces would change, but the characters would most likely always remain the same. So, the next time you're tempted by jealousy, just remember that someone else wants your easy job.

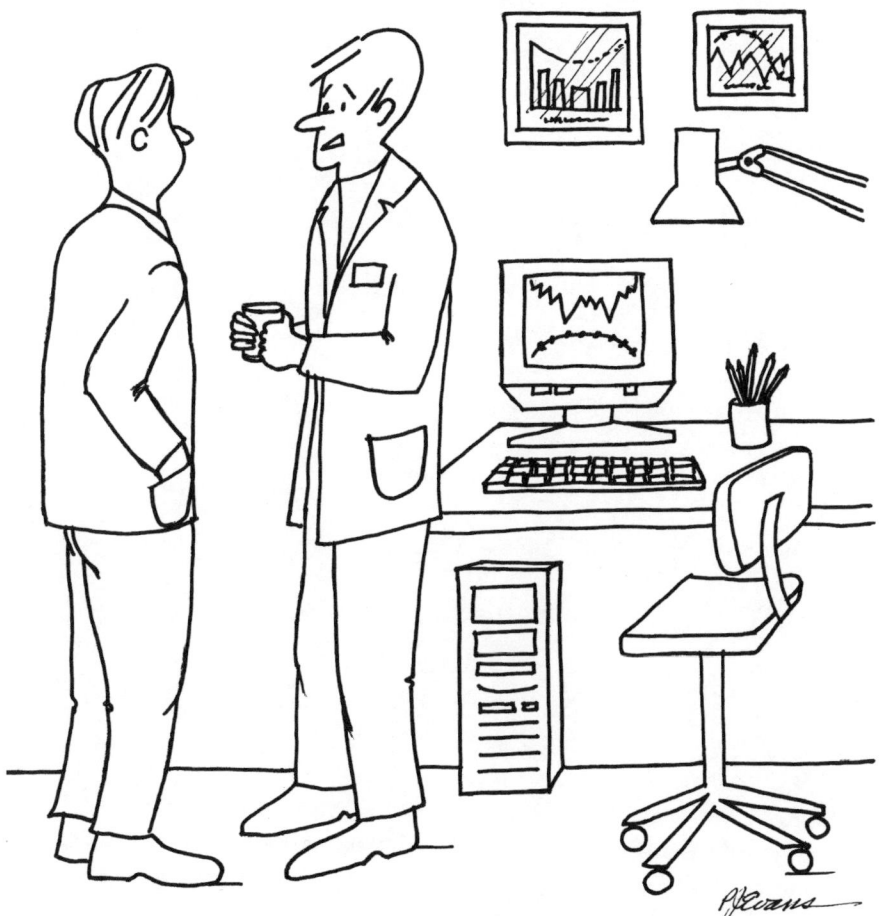

"No, really, I'm telling you that computer hates me."

NEW YAWK, NEW YAWK

Dexter Hunt, BA, EMT-P

Every so often, a kid gets to fulfill a fantasy, perhaps involving a journey, castles and a dragon or two. Could one ask for anything more?

I have to credit Brooklyn paramedic David Spiro with the idea for my most recent fantasy. "Why don't we switch EMS systems for a week or so?" David proposed. Sure, I thought, I'd be willing to give up clean air, drinkable water and a low crime rate for a 1-week gig in the most populous city on the North American continent. David was asking me to leave Idaho for a city with 30 times the population density, four times the violent crime and, even more scary, 35 times the number of lawyers. It sounded great. How could I say no?

New York City is big. You feel the energy the moment you step onto its streets. It has culture, art and an endless variety of crime and humanity. On my first subway ride, I found more cultural diversity than in the entire state of Idaho.

Before leaving home, I had received an extensive subway-safety briefing. "Stay out of the subways after 7 p.m.—and for God's sake, stay away from the edge of the loading platform," Dave had cautioned. You have to maintain a distance from the edge, he informed me, because people here actually push others off the platform and into the paths of oncoming trains. Those victims unfortunate enough to land in front of the train are either electrocuted on the charged third rail or crushed by the train. On occasion, a victim is pinned between the side of the train and the loading platform. He then becomes what's referred to as a "space case," suspended with a normally lethal injury.

The Day Shift

7 a.m. to 3 p.m.—Putting on a bullet-resistant vest is a pleasant reminder that we're entering a war zone. One of my passions is scene safety and survival tactics. After 15 years in law enforcement, I've examined the gap between what EMTs learn in class and what they face on the streets. As a result, I've developed safety strategies that have worked in every setting, and I'm eager to try them in this high-risk community. I'm happy to report they worked.

Working out of St. Mary's Hospital in Brooklyn, I experience the Bedford-Stuyvesant (Bed-Stuy) area of 250,000 people. It's also known as "Little Beirut." One of the street mottoes for Bed-Stuy EMS providers is "Give us 2 minutes and we'll give you a shooting." Sadly, the shooting is often in the direction of EMS personnel.

The sound of automatic weapons fired across alleys as fights play out among the numerous crack dealers is intimidating, but I'm grateful these aggressive "businessmen" haven't learned how to properly lay down a field of fire. Consider the mortality rate if they actually took the time to practice, aim and use selective fire! While not as dramatic as an Uzi spraying down an alley, a high-power rifle with a scope will kill just as effectively.

But New York's calls really aren't different from those received in other EMS systems. Patients are patients, regardless of their city or dwelling. The sheer volume and constant pressure on the overall NYC EMS system, however, are overwhelming. In a year, NYC EMS and its voluntary EMS units will answer about 1.2 million calls. Keeping up with them is like trying to fix a ruptured aortic aneurysm with a Calvin and Hobbes Band-Aid. Sadly, 45% of these calls are either hoaxes, fakes or vanishing patients.

We log onto the CAD computer as 35 Victor (tirty-foive vic, in New Yorkese). New York runs both BLS and ALS ambulances. In the local EMS jargon, a call is a *job*, an ambulance is a *bus* and a station is an *outpost*. (It's interesting that the U.S. Cavalry called its frontier forts exactly that: outposts.)

We respond to a "difficulty breathing" in a third-floor apartment. All calls are run in the emergency mode to and from the scene. The 35 members of the family and friends live in a three-room complex. Dave and his partner, Tony Morgan, take the history.

Reprinted with permission from Emergency Medical Services, © 1992; 21(3):22, 26, 28. Edited from the original.

The patient is a 25-year-old female with a 6-month-old cough. Her mother died last week of tuberculosis. She's Haitian and speaks no English. There are so many different languages, cultures and dialects here that it's often difficult to communicate with your patients.

During the ride to the hospital, the driver of a 10-ton truck decides that the best evasion strategy is to put the truck in reverse and back into us while we're running the code. The front of the ambulance caves in. We now have to call for another unit to transport the patient. I briefly entertain the thought of putting on a cervical collar, rolling on the ground and claiming a severe spinal-cord injury. I then remember that every spinal-cord patient I take in gets a Foley catheter. I decide to stay quiet and continue waking upright.

A new call comes in immediately, followed by another and yet another. It's difficult to run emergency calls in a town where the citizens actively try to get you to slam on your brakes and double-parking is a way of life.

Later, we pull into Kings County Hospital, an area trauma center. If not *the* busiest trauma center in the world, it's one of them. Bed after bed is filled with trauma—basic, advanced and terminal. The patient load is so heavy that it's not unusual to wait several hours before turning over your patient to the overworked ED staff. The waiting rooms are bulging. Patients sit in double rows of chairs, down one wall and up the next. If you didn't know better, you'd think they were waiting for tickets to a Rolling Stones concert. Field crews check their on-board CRT screens and note hospital after hospital beginning voluntary diversions. Ambulances with more patients are in holding patterns.

Major incidents that are rare in many parts of the United States happen with regularity here. On my first day, Manhattan loses all electrical power from a substation problem, and EMS helps hand-ventilate patients at area hospitals. On another morning, two buses collide, injuring 21 people. The EMS system quickly absorbs and treats these multicasualty incidents in an efficient manner. These are professional rescuers.

In spite of all of the pressures, field crews continually back up and assist each other, call after call. It's common for one car to take a call for another car that's been getting hammered. And so it goes, call after call, hour after hour. This routine is repeated day after day in New York, as well as in other large cities' EMS systems. EMTs and paramedics attempt to stay in the field and beat the burnout clock that ticks away.

"No Apologies, No Problem . . ."

There's currently an increased awareness of critical incident stress (CIS) and its devastating sequelae. One of its major contributors is injury to fellow EMS workers. As we finish our long shift, with more than a few frustrating calls, what's left of the endogenous epinephrine in our adrenal glands is squirted into our bodies when word reaches us that EMS personnel were left broken and bleeding by correctional officers at Rikers Island. It's bad enough when the public enjoys open-hunting season on EMTs, but it's an outrage when law-enforcement officers participate in aggravated assaults on EMS personnel. No apologies, no problem. New York EMS personnel are used to this kind of treatment. They work on the streets, providing care to the sick and injured, and yet they're not even considered a uniformed service; sanitation employees *are*. EMS workers have to wear green; so do sanitation workers. The starting salary for a paramedic is $27,000 a year; sanitation workers start at $30,000.

The Nerve Center

David takes me on a tour of the communications/dispatch center. This impressive building contains the hardware and human resources that act as the nerve center for EMS in New York City. It's one of the few buildings on the block not covered with graffiti. In New York, graffiti is used like glue; it holds many buildings together.

Dispatchers are an important link in the provision of care in any EMS system. New York is no exception. Someone has to answer the 1.2 million calls for help. The volume of telephone activity is amazing. The dispatch center handles an EMS call every 2 *seconds*. After selectively screening and prioritizing the level of response, the dispatchers maintain the direction of 150 ambulances that are on duty at any given time. They do it very well.

Dispatchers are the lifeblood of any busy EMS system. Without them, EMTs/paramedics would be without direction and support. How would it be if, for once, dispatchers were given some of the creature comforts that the field staff enjoys? What would it be like if someone designed a dispatch center that provided a good work environment? Most dispatch centers are designed for security first, dispatchers second. This means they're located in dark basements with stagnant air or in the center of a building, without any windows. Most dispatchers would love to see the outside to know there really is a world out there.

Unfortunately, the design theory behind dispatch centers is that terrorists or other malcontents might have access to the dispatchers. Believe me, it's easier to blow up the transmission towers. Does anyone actually think an EMS center would last for any length of time under a direct assault by a heavily armed terrorist group?

35 Victor handles a total of 34 calls over 24 hours, including six shootings, three stabbings, an ambulance accident and a bullet hole through the left front fender. After an 8-hour shift with 12 calls, a shower is necessary. It washes off the humanity of the streets and the dirt of the day's calls.

My time in New York ends far too quickly. My memories and impressions will last a long time. NYC EMS is a system of size, volume and caring—one that has so much tradition and camaraderie that it's exciting. Watching the crews of St. Mary's and other EMS personnel work under the volume and adversity, and the dirt and violence of the projects, makes me proud to do what we all do: take care of patients. My deepest thanks to the EMS providers in "New Yawk" who allowed me to experience their world.

LEARNING EXPERIENCES

Renea Akin, MHS, PT

One recent evening, my 11-year-old son walked up to my husband and asked, "Dad, can I borrow your saw?" Those, I thought to myself, are words to stop the heart of any parent.

While holding my breath and awaiting my husband's cautious reply, I started thinking about lines my students have used that would stop the heart of any instructor. For example, before our often-zealous charges go out into the clinic, I have learned to remind them that, although their clinical instructor may not be carrying out a task in exactly the same manner in which we covered the material in class, the clinical instructor is not necessarily wrong.

This year, however, I guess I got busy and forgot.

This year, I noticed one of my students who does not usually volunteer for class discussion appeared eager to share her experience with her classmates. I congratulated myself on my expertise in facilitating communication and quickly called on her. My enthusiasm turned to dismay as she began her tale: "I noticed during my clinical that they weren't doing so-and-so the way you taught us, so I told my clinician you said. . . ."

I reached for my roll of TUMS and, in my mind, began composing an apology letter to the clinician. I'm beginning to think I should change my outgoing voice mail message to include a version of the note sent home by my son's kindergarten teacher that read, "I won't believe everything they say about you if you don't believe everything they say about me."

My students are consistently creative, if not always accurate. It also appears that they have also been told somewhere in their academic careers never to leave a test question unanswered. That has to be the reason one dutiful student wrote on an examination that the abbreviation "ORIF" stands for "Operating Room is Full." To this day, when I come across the abbreviation ORIF, I envision rows of gurneys lined up in a hallway outside an operating room, each holding a silent, expectant patient.

Reprinted from PT: Magazine of Physical Therapy, © 1999; 7(2):84, with permission of the APTA and the author. Edited from the original.

Although not all students complete all reading assignments on time, most do attempt to keep up the pretense of having read the material. One student who had been playing this game blew it midway through the section on neurology. She left her neuro book in the lab—still tightly wrapped in plastic. She assured me, however, that, although she had not yet had time to open the book, she was sleeping with it every night. Does learning occur by osmosis, I wonder? Should I offer her some TUMS?

I learn all sorts of things during lab check-offs, including what kinds of mistakes I might have made. Students who enter a PT or PTA education program are usually high achievers academically, and they are unaccustomed to being wrong. Therefore, they are often astonished during lab check-offs when they realize they have been practicing treatment techniques in error. This is evidenced by such responses as "You mean the 6 to 8 layers of toweling go between the patient and hot pack? I thought they were there to insulate the hot pack and keep the heat next to the patient!" TUMS come in different flavors, you know.

Even though those lab check-offs are stressful, they allow mistakes to be made in such a way that the only real injury is to the ego of the student or instructor.

And if you're wondering about my son, he was allowed to borrow the saw. He's in the basement building a machine designed to shoot tennis balls for folks like me who need extra practice. Of course, as with my students, he'll require some supervision before he's ready to use the saw on his own. I wonder what my students will create if they're given the right tools?

ASK SIRENHEAD

Sirenhead

Dear Sirenhead: We keep leaving equipment on scenes. It's embarrassing, but in one week, we left behind an oxygen resuscitator and a portable suction. Is this a common problem? Please don't print our names.
—*"Andy" and "Mike," Via Internet*

My 4-year-old has the same problem with his toys, but hey, no one's perfect. Here's my suggestion—after you clear the ED, always, always, go back for the equipment you left. It's foolproof. If you have to go back enough times, you'll stop leaving it. It cured me. My partner and I actually had to break into a house once to get our drug box back. The whole family was at the hospital, and we weren't going to tell the safety-pin-counting supervisor we were KO'd. So we found a loose window, fed the dog a doughnut and crawled in and got the box. Another time, a bunch of cops made us bring them a pizza before they would tell us where our monitor was. I've even had to go back to people's bedrooms after we cleared and look in the bed sheets for the portable radio. Do that a few times, and you won't leave anything behind—not even a bad smell. In the meantime, if you get a call and discover you've lost an essential piece of equipment (like the stretcher), keep cool. Good medics know how to punt.

Dear Sirenhead: Where I work we have seniority shift bidding. As the new guy, I don't think it's fair because I always have to work nights and weekends. What would you do?—*B.R., New York*

You'd love to work with me—I hate day shifts, makes my blood pressure go up working when the brass is around. I don't like Richie Cunninghams nosing around trying to find something to manage. It probably won't surprise you to learn I like my independence. One of the reasons I'm in EMS is, if you work it right, you can have a lot of freedom. Of course, if you work the off shifts, you got to be

Reprinted with permission from JEMS: Journal of Emergency Medical Services, © 1997; 22(8):104.

resourceful and manage yourself. You've got to be innovative, figure out how you're going to fix the stretcher in the middle of the night, and forget about whining to someone up the ladder.

Besides, you get better calls at night. Maybe it's the added challenge of popping lines in the dark or maybe it's because the yuppie, cell-phone-hugging BMW drivers are home in bed. I'm not sure why, but I like dark streets, red lights slapping up-side a dark building, and the midnight weirdos at the Castle when you stop to pick up a bag of sliders. Even if you don't do much on a night shift, when you go home, you've got that good tired feeling—like you did something important. When I work days, I get off and feel agitated—like I need to go do some real work, and that's when my wife hits me up to fix the toilet or haul the laundry downstairs. Who wants to do that when you come home? An empty house suits me just fine for a few hours. Then I get to spend some time with my kid before hitting the streets again.

Fair? Of course it's not. Ask the guy who ate the dashboard if life is fair. Ask the skinny lady with cancer if life is fair. When you stop expecting fairness, you start living. Take advantage of the schedule, make it work for you and stop whining.

PROSTATES AND OTHER TOUCHY SUBJECTS

Thomas W. O'Connor, PharmD, MBA

Can a young female pharmacist talk to me about my old prostate? The answer, of course, is "yes," but I have some real sensitivities and concerns... not about my prostate... but about her. My first concern is that she may not be able to appreciate the psychological trauma associated with diseases that strike at the heart of my sexual competencies. My second concern is: "I'm not comfortable discussing sexual issues with a young pharmacist. A gender difference makes it all that much more difficult."

Now I know I should be more clinical, more objective, more receptive, but I'm not. Maybe if I had female health care professionals as I grew up, I'd be more comfortable. But I didn't. I'm old fashioned, but that's how I feel. Now I can "hear" young women pharmacists saying "get a life," "get over it," and/or "why is your prostate more sensitive than my ovaries as a topic of discussion." I don't have an answer for you, but you're the health care professional who's supposed to understand. Do I need to have a rational basis for my feelings before they're considered valid? I think not.

You're going to have to deal with my insecurities with pharmacists of the opposite sex. Sorry that I haven't matured in my attitudes, but if you can accept that, you are then in a position to help me get past them.

First, show me that you're comfortable with the subject. Nothing makes me more embarrassed than when I embarrass someone else. Demonstrate, up front, that you are ready, willing, and able to address my prostate problem professionally and objectively. And remember, I'm watching for body language that shows me you can handle the topic. That's not a blush I see... is it?

Then you need to show me that you can speak my language. I already know that you're young. Don't let your manner of speech make you seem younger. Try to keep the "likes" and "ya knows" out of your discussion with me. If I hear you say: "your prostate is like bigger, and it like presses on your urethra ya know," I'll feel as though I'm talking to a little girl.

Another helpful technique is to use simple analogies that move the discussion away from sexual

Reprinted with permission from Pharmacy Times, © 1997; 63(10):16. Edited from the original.

connotations. You may want to use plumbing, electric, and construction analogies to make your teaching points. I can relate to them and I'm comfortable with them. Anything to get away from direct references to my prostate. Plumbing works well for urogenital and cardiac diseases. Nervous disorders are obviously electrical problems. Bones and connective tissue disorders are construction problems. Teaching through analogies is a real art form, and you'll want to practice to get good at it.

You also need to show me that you relate to my problem. If you tell me that you have family members, friends, or even acquaintances with the same problem, then I know that you're at least sensitive to my concerns. I'd just hate to be the first person to discuss this issue with you.

Certainly you have to show me that you "know your stuff." I expect that you can easily discuss lifestyle changes, drug therapy, monitoring, and dealing with complications without your class notes. Here's where you show me you didn't just study to pass the exam.

You also need to respect my privacy during the discussion. Counseling areas, quiet conversation, and an awareness of others around us are all appreciated more than you know. It makes no sense to help me get over my embarrassment with you just to turn around and embarrass me in front of a third party. If we can't talk in the pharmacy, then please call me at home.

Finally, keep my problem to yourself. Don't make me the center of your recount of the day to friends. Don't discuss me with uninvolved colleagues. Bottom line . . . keep my trust in you. That's the maturity I'm looking for. It's the essence of the professionalism that you value so highly. Maintain it even when you're not in the pharmacy. It's not an act. It's an attitude.

Now I know that we've discussed this through the eyes of a male baby boomer. We could just as easily have titled the article: "Can a Young Male Pharmacist Talk to Me About My Old Ovaries?" Nothing would have changed. I'd just have more difficulty writing in the first person singular. By the way, all references to diseases were hypothetical . . . honest.

SO HERE'S ANOTHER VALENTINE'S DAY

Kathy Nephew
Maribeth Leahy

So here's another Valentine's Day,
We wish you happiness in every way.
And just to show you we understand,
Here's a poem from our own hand.

Your day began in such a fright,
You worked all day and half the night.
Fluoro at 8:00, it was no drag,
There were ten holes in the enema bag.

From BE to GI you go,
What might happen, you'll never know.
No time to waste, no time to spare,
You're needed here, you're needed there.

A ton of x-rays by your side,
These are the times you'd like to hide.
But there's so many to be done,
And you're only on number one.

All day long at the viewbox you stare,
People coming at you from everywhere.
Stacks of film flung on a cart,
Half the folders are falling apart.

Alas, dear doctors, your day is complete,
It's time to relax your aching feet.
We think it's a wonder, you're still alive,
Let's hope tomorrow you will survive.

Reprinted with permission from Radiologic Technology, © 1985; 56(3):178.

AN EMS CHRISTMAS

Sheila Drazic

'Twas the night before Christmas and all through our town,
Ambulances sat quietly—call volume was down.
Dispatchers and medics, without any calls,
All settled cozily within station walls.
The city grew silent as the night grew deep;
My partner and I settled in for some sleep.
But no sooner dreaming in our beds were we,
When dispatch awoke us, crying, "Hurry! Code 3!"
The call had come in for an MVA;
Some nutcase, claimed he'd hit Santa's sleigh!
"Head trauma," we thought, as we gathered our gear,
"Or maybe a drunk driver—it's that time of year."
As we raced to the scene with our sirens and lights,
We hoped for the best, tonight of all nights.
We had no idea we were in for a surprise
And, on our arrival, couldn't believe our own eyes.
I said to my partner, "This must be a trick!
"That man in the ditch just *can't* be Saint Nick!"
A smashed-up sleigh! Toys thrown far and near!
And off to the side, a group of reindeer!
The driver of the car, with a bump on his head
Was crying and told us he wished he was dead.
"Oh, why did I have that one extra beer?
"Now I've killed Santa—no Christmas this year!"
By now we'd decided that this was too strange,
So we tried to call backup, but were out of range.
"No radio contact," to my partner I said,
"I'll check out that one while you dress this one's head."
I approached the man in the ditch with great care.
He was dressed so oddly—he gave me a scare.
He wore a red suit and a strange kind of hat.
I thought to myself, "Who dresses like that?"
Then he opened his eyes and said, "Do not fear.
"Just please help me up—I must catch my reindeer."
I said, "The reindeer are fine, but stay where you are.
"You've taken a pretty hard hit from that car."
I didn't want to leave him, so I let out a holler:
"We're gonna need backboard, head blocks and collar!"
As we worked, the man cried, "No! Please don't strap me down.
"I have toys to deliver all over town!
"All of the children tonight are depending on me
"To get their presents under the Christmas tree."
"I'm sorry," I told him, as I shook my head sadly,
"You're going to the hospital—you've been hurt too badly."
He looked up at me and wiped away a tear
And told me, "Then *you* must bring the Christmas presents this year!"
"Visit every child's home in this town?" asked I.
"Sir, you must think I can make an ambulance fly!"
I thought I had made a serious blunder,
For his eyes grew steely, and his voice was like thunder.
"Now Dasher, now Dancer, now Prancer and Vixen,
"Come Comet and Cupid and Donner and Blitzen!
"Hitch onto that truck and take to the sky
"For tonight, indeed, an ambulance *will* fly!"
I just shook my head as we loaded him in,
Then climbed in the cab and I just had to grin.
There were the reindeer, all in a row,
In front of the truck as if ready to go.
"That's cute," I thought. "I'll just go around."
But then they took off and our wheels left the ground!
Away we went, up over the trees,
Sailing along as light as a breeze.
We touched down on rooftops, delivering toys,
Dropping gifts for good little girls and boys.
We stopped briefly in the hospital's ambulance bay
And wheeled him to the ED—and hoped he'd stay.
"We'll call in report later," we said on our way.
"This man's turned our ambulance into a sleigh!"
Then off we flew, all through the night,
Delivering toys till the dawn's first light.
Finally, at our station, we headed down,

Reprinted with permission from Emergency Medical Services, ©1995; 24(11):22.

Both of us happy to be on the ground.
Dispatch was mad, but the more we explained,
The less they believed and the more they looked pained.
So we sat in our quarters—boy, were we in trouble!
We turned on the news and perked up on the double.

As TV crews interviewed people around town,
It seemed that some very strange things had gone down.
Tire tracks were found on a rooftop or two
And children said, "This year, Santa wore blue!"
I grinned at my partner and said, "It's no mystery!
"This Christmas will go down in EMS history!"

THE TECH WHO MOOED AT A SURGEON

Michael Ramsey, PhD, CLS(NCA), CLSpH(NCA)

Dr. Maynard was undoubtedly the best surgeon in our hospital. Some staff members considered him one of the best general surgeons in the region. Unfortunately, although Dr. Maynard was a superb surgeon and treated his patients royally, few hospital employees could stand to work with him. Abrasive was one of the kinder terms used to describe him. He was not above reprimanding other staff members in front of patients or coworkers. He often used the term "incompetent" to describe other staff members, including surgeons. When his mother needed surgery, Dr. Maynard took the case rather than let another surgeon operate on her.

Dr. Maynard could have earned the respect of everyone in our institution if his temper had not been so fearsome. No one in the medical lab had ever seen anyone stand up to Dr. Maynard. This was before the arrival of Wesley.

Wesley was an excellent medical technologist. He turned out good work, followed lab policy to the letter, and treated everyone with respect. But Wesley was different. His personality was, to say the least, "unique." Although no one in the lab actually got to know Wesley, we knew he had a supportive family, was highly recommended by his former employer, and was eccentric. When the Chief of Pathology discussed something with Wesley, Wesley could often be seen making a paper-clip necklace or a paper airplane. Everyone was amused by Wesley and enjoyed working with him. Then Wesley met Dr. Maynard.

Wesley and I were working in hematology when we received a call from the ER for some blood work. Wesley agreed to go. When he arrived, Wesley was told that Dr. Maynard wanted a CBC, SMAC, and a bleeding panel. Wesley entered the cubicle to collect the specimens. Since the patient had no identification band and was semicomatose, Wesley asked Dr. Maynard to identify the patient. Dr. Maynard, who was listening to the patient's heart, abruptly took off his stethoscope and shouted at Wesley for interrupting his examination, calling him a fool and threatening to have him fired if he ever disturbed him again. Wesley just stood there, mute. The nurse who overheard the outburst quickly identified the patient. After Wesley collected the specimens, he paused at the door.

"And what are you waiting for? Get those damn specimens to the lab!" shouted Dr. Maynard.

With that, Wesley looked at Dr. Maynard in the face and said "Moo-o-o-o!" just like a cow, then calmly walked out.

The nurse said that Dr. Maynard turned such a deep red color she thought he was going to catch fire.

Wesley returned to the lab and began to process the specimens. He said nothing of the incident to

Reprinted with permission from Clinical Laboratory Science, © 1994; 7(4):196.

anyone. Two minutes later Dr. Maynard arrived and went straight to the office of Chief of Pathology. Although there was a thick glass window between the office and the lab, everyone could hear them.

Dr. Maynard (pointing at Wesley): "I want that idiot fired!"

Chief: "And why do you want him fired?"

Dr. Maynard: "He mooed at me in front of a patient!"

Chief: "Mooed? Like a cow?"

Dr. Maynard: "Yeah! Some people are so disrespectful!"

Chief: "Well, I'll agree that is highly irregular behavior, but I'm not sure it is grounds for termination. I'll consult the hospital employee policy manual and get back to you."

The Chief of Pathology, who had been the recipient of many of Dr. Maynard's verbal outbursts, could not help smiling at the situation. Realizing that he was getting nowhere, Dr. Maynard stormed out of the lab. As the Chief discussed the matter with the section supervisor, they saw Wesley sitting at his post nearby wearing a pair of toy glasses, a fake nose, and mustache, giving him the appearance of Groucho Marx. Dr. Maynard probably never forgot the "mooing incident." He was rarely seen in the lab again, which pleased the lab personnel. What happened to Wesley? Nothing, really. The Chief counseled him about his behavior and told him to avoid Dr. Maynard in the future. Wesley still receives excellent performance ratings and annual merit pay raises.

Five years after leaving the hospital, I ran into a former coworker who had worked with Wesley and me. She told me Wesley was still working at the hospital and was still as efficient and "unique" as ever. She also said that Wesley had become a staff hero. One day she had overheard two physicians who had noticed Wesley walking across the room. One physician asked the other, "Hey, isn't that the guy from the lab who mooed at Dr. Maynard? Wow! Those med techs have guts!"

THE PERTURBED RATTLER

Greg Nelson, EMT-P

A paramedic learns he must work hard to get a head in this world.

I once had a partner and roommate named Les, who spent all of his leisure time attending classes at the local college. I applauded his efforts—after all, anyone who works as a full-time EMT and goes to school deserves applause. Even more important, this gave me some solo time at home.

Les was an OK sort of guy, with only the usual smattering of bad habits. He occasionally left food on the stereo or strange women unattended in the living room. I soon learned to tolerate his misconception that I was interested in his school work. I didn't put up a fuss when he shorted out our electrical power with a science project, and I even managed to remain calm when he stored a ready-for-dissection cat in the refrigerator. But I eventually had to draw the line when his interest turned to psychology.

Les found in me a wealth of material worthy of study. You might think I'd be flattered, but after a few weeks of his analyzing everything from my handwriting to the time I spent in the bathroom it grew tiresome. One night, I made a gross error and told him I was uncomfortable around snakes. This regrettable disclosure started a very complicated chain of events.

For several days after my admission, Les conducted a series of experiments. At various times

Reprinted with permission from Emergency Medical Services, © 1993; 22(11):61–62.

and locations, I'd find a realistic rubber snake or even a live garter snake hidden in unlikely spots. Invariably, Les would be there to record my response. The experiments stopped after I was surprised by a garden snake hidden in the dishwasher and Les received several stitches that left a barbecue-spatula-shaped scar.

It all came to a head late one Saturday night when Les and I were at work. We were dispatched to, of all things, a snakebite. All the way to the scene, I could feel Les studying me, and I resolved, just this once, to show no signs of fear.

Upon our arrival, we found our patient—a grizzly old man—standing stoically in the road, in no apparent distress. As I approached him, he volunteered that he'd been bitten by a "rattler" and couldn't get his pickup started. He gestured down to his right leg, and I noted that he had cut and bled the wound in the Old West tradition.

I looked around as inconspicuously as possible and, not spotting a snake, decided to help the patient into the ambulance. We were just about to go on our merry way when, off in the distance, there came the cry of a small voice.

"Wait! Y'all want this?" the youthful voice called out.

Fearing what "this" was, I hoped no one else had heard him and urged Les to hurry up and drive. But, alas, the body caught up with the voice, and a teenage boy stood at the back door of the ambulance with a large paper sack in hand. He was a little winded and, after a moment to compose himself, asked, "You wanna take the snake? I killed it with a shovel."

The pride in his voice annoyed me, but not as much as the smirk on my partner's face. We'd learned in our training to always take the offending reptile to the hospital, if possible. I was so disgusted, in fact, that my usual grip on good sense left me.

"Sure, just set it down there," I said.

It was almost worth seeing Les gasp in surprise and trade his grimace for a puzzled expression, tinged with respect.

Off we drove into the night, and I concentrated on treating the victim, even though he kept repeating, "I don't need any of that stuff—just take me to the hospital."

It was right after dutifully applying the lymphatic tourniquets and starting the IV that I heard it: a high buzz that made my insides quiver and sweat roll from my forehead. Hoping it was merely a hallucination, but fearing the worst, I carefully turned to gaze at the sack. My anxiety proved justified. The rattler, though mortally wounded, was rising up out of the bag.

I once saw a show on PBS about snakes, during which the narrator explained that reptiles are devoid of emotion and totally dependent upon reflex. Sure, that sounded good on TV, but let me tell you something: This particular snake was *pissed*. A gaping wound that hadn't quite severed its head was evidently the reason behind the perturbed expression on its pointed face, and I was clearly the target of its vengeance.

Retreating to the far corner of the ambulance, I screamed loud enough to drown out the siren.

"Stop this @!*&#$ing ambulance, you stupid %$$#!" I yelled.

Les, always one to respond quickly, stood up on the brake pedal, causing snake, paramedic, equipment and patient to be thrown violently against the forward bulkhead.

As the rig came to a rest—and before the snake could get its bearings—I ran out the back door faster than a bullet leaves a gun.

Standing on the side of the interstate, searching for bite marks, I considered a career change. I was just beginning to wonder about what to do next when my forgotten patient exited the ambulance. He made quite a picture: O_2 mask hanging around his neck and carrying his own IV bag in his right hand. But it was his left hand that caught my attention. Grasping it by the tail, he held the still-twitching 5½' diamondback rattlesnake. Calmly, and with only minor effort, he placed his boot on the snake's half-severed head and pulled. The head popped off, but the rest of the snake's body continued to jump and writhe.

The man stepped forward and handed me the snake, right at the precise moment Les was rounding the corner of the ambulance. My arm seemed to act on its own, or perhaps it was guided by fate, but as soon as my hand closed on the dying reptile, I flung it with all my might. It had to be divine intervention, but for years after the incident I'd be accused of aiming—and so help me, I didn't intend for the snake to become wrapped around my partner's neck. Les, unaware that the dreaded serpent lacked a head or fangs, panicked. He began flailing about, trying desperately to dislodge the fast-expiring rattler.

In retrospect, it was quite a sight, worthy of a Stephen King film. The ambulance's strobes caused Les's frantic arm-waving and exaggerated dance steps to be frozen in time for an instant. Realizing that his relatively stationary panic was ineffective, Les elected to try running, and off he went into the night. Just as he achieved top speed, a tree interrupted his flight, and that's where my patient and I found him—face up and out cold, still in the embrace of the irked, but now definitely dead, rattler.

We must have made quite a picture for the highway patrol guys—the patient apparently healthy, the paramedic laughing hysterically, and the EMT suffering from a slight concussion and wearing a snake. We explained over and over again why the ambulance was blocking the road.

We eventually made it to the hospital, but we left the snake on the highway shoulder, just in case anyone didn't believe it was a rattler and wanted to check it out—we'd be glad to provide directions on where to find it.

As for Les and me, we remained friends, even though he sometimes got annoyed with me over my newfound interest in scientific experiments. I never tired of watching his reaction to a well-placed rubber snake.

SO WE THINK WE ARE UNIQUE...

Mary Jenkins

Occupational therapists are practitioners. We interact directly with clients. That interaction is intended to be helpful; therefore, occupational therapy can be defined as one of the helping professions. Yet what are, or can we identify, the distinctive characteristics of our particular profession? A useful illuminant is the question: how are occupational therapists unique?

Recent research highlights some interesting points. To the question "In your opinion, what if anything is unique about occupational therapy?" the array of answers, rather than being a guide to the uniqueness of the profession, attests to its ever-wide spectrum. To quote a diplomate, "I think what's unique about occupational therapy is we do a bit of everything." The 16 different responses given extend along a continuum from "I don't think there's anything unique about occupational therapy" to "Everything is unique about occupational therapy."

So what is meant by "unique"? As aptly stated by an administrator, "If you're unique, you should be standing out and others should know your role and the boundaries of your role." However, this is not the case. We, ourselves, do not know. Perhaps we are as bemused as the person who replied, "The name, it doesn't convey what occupational therapy does." This is an argument which can be used by many professions today. Very few disciplines hold true to the original meaning of their name; as one doctor interviewed remarked, "Nurses will do anything except nursing." Professional development does dictate that changes will occur. If we were only to deal with what and how we began, our need would long since have been dissipated.

It will be no surprise to any occupational therapist that among the most prevalent evidence of our uniqueness is our holistic approach. However, as noted by an educator, "We glibly say that we are the only holistic profession and it's not true. And anyway, doctors, physiotherapists, social workers would argue the same thing." Of equal standing is our functional aspect. A speech and language therapist describes us as "the ones who have this whole

Reprinted with permission of the author and British Journal of Occupational Therapy, © 1993; 56(1):1. Edited from the original.

total overview of the person." This image of the functional therapist is one that other professionals and clients identify readily with us. "You're one of the people who is genuinely appreciated by the patients because you bring a practical aspect to their life."

If this is the case, then why is it that we do not acknowledge it as our uniqueness and build on it? Educators prefer to think that "activity" is our uniqueness. This notion of activity is also shared by assistants but for quite different reasons.

The most eloquent evocation of our uniqueness came from a client's comment: "I don't know but it's something that no-one else applies. It moves slightly outside the medical treatment. It moves you into society." This not only exposes the value of occupational therapy but also acknowledges its historical foundations in medicine, with which we are still and should be involved, and the societal elements of participation and membership, with which we are inevitably involved.

ABSOLUTELY FLABULOUS

Colleen Wedderburn Tate

It's that time of year again—sun, sea, cellulite and skin cancer. Most of us vigorously pursue the first two and try to avoid the last. The ultimate goal is a glowingly healthy body, preferably without blemish, toned to within an inch of its life, and fit to be seen in all the right places.

To this end, the fitness industry is (to coin a phrase) coining it. We are exhorted to avoid nasties such as dimpled thighs, arms and backs, and to treat the sun with extreme prejudice. Anything that might lead to the Body You Have Always Wanted is actively promoted. Keeping fit is a universal goal. And that is official.

The Health Education Authority is seeking couch potatoes—those subversive enemies of a "healthy lifestyle" who believe that exercise of any kind, other than opening and closing the mouth at regular intervals to eat unhealthy foods, is strictly non-U.

The HEA's three-year programme "encourages England to become Active for Life." But wait. Apparently, "sweating and panting" are out (bang go my Tuesday mornings), but "doing enough activity to get warm and slightly out of breath" is in. Oh goody. And how English. None of this messy heavy-breathing stuff, just something nice and genteel. Ultimately, "we [the HEA] want to help people lead a more *active* life [their italics]—not tell them to take more exercise."

But if the HEA does not get you, your employer might. Some companies, and the government, want a healthy productive workforce because this will cut costs. These so-called workplace wellness programmes originated in the USA where, as it lacks a national healthcare system, a significant proportion of company profit is eaten up by health care benefits.

So is this another case of over-there-will-soon-be-over-here? Not quite. People who are fit and well do not suffer from "presenteeism," meaning turning up for work but going at half-throttle. Also, if you feel well, you feel confident, friendly, and are less likely to pick up bugs.

Having said that, workplace wellness programmes are no substitute for treating employees like human beings. Employees who fear for their jobs and are in constant danger of being allocated mushroom status will not benefit much from a fitness programme that does not include psychological muscle-boosters such as "please," "thank you," and "well done."

Neither will people thank the boss if they lose out in the promotion stakes because the real business of the organisation is done in a wine bar, not over the handlebars of a stationary cycle.

Reproduced by kind permission of Nursing Times, where this article first appeared, July 10, 1996; 92(28):52. Edited from the original.

If you still feel a little nip of fear about the contents of your next inhouse staff newsletter, breathe out slowly and murmur "Pleasure Revenge." From the people who brought you fudge-flavoured popcorn, and Faith Popcorn (a person not a religious fast-food), Pleasure Revenge is wresting our bodies from the evils of aerobics, little piles of green leaves on a large plate and the other iniquities peddled by those people for whom the word fat was an obscene word, at least while there was money to be made.

Seekers of the Pleasure Revenge path indulge in such wickedness as smoking cigars, eating red meat and cinnamon buns. Ms Popcorn, who is a "trendspotter," claims Pleasure Revenge will become the dominant trend of the 1990s. But as the decade is nearly over, the UK will, once again, miss out. Can't say I'm sorry.

Like a healthy lifestyle, Pleasure Revenge requires money—to pay for cigars, steak, expensive cognacs, and, undoubtedly, clothes to go with this new trend. The people who really need to improve their physical health have few resources to do so. If you have a warm home, a change of clothing, a GP, some food, and are on fairly amicable terms with your neighbour, that is a minimum base from which to hop into a healthy life. But isn't it strange that, as soon as the hoi polloi get with it down at the gym, the trendsetters are off elsewhere.

I once spotted a book called *Flatten Your Stomach—For Women Over 35*. It said that with a flat stomach I would be more confident. Like Pleasure Revenge, or exhortations to get fit, those with confidence don't need the books. A flat stomach may mean clothes fit better but confidence comes from somewhere else.

The British, thank goodness, are healthily sceptical of trends and happily discuss the dangers of a high-fat diet over scampi and chips in the pub. Personally, I am off to the gym for some heavy panting and dubious conversation. You see, I am getting ready to stay out of the sun, and the costumes required for this are far more revealing than any bikini.

My cellulite is recovering nicely, and will be gloriously enhanced by the graceful raising and lowering of each arm, at the end of which will be a frosted glass of pink fizzing stuff. Have a coolly simmering summer. And watch out for low-flying trendspotters.

FIRST PERSON

Brendan Smith, EMT-P

I'm as guilty as you are. We all do it, and sometimes we're not even aware of it. It's almost a requirement of the profession, although we certainly didn't learn it in EMT school. What is it? The telling of war stories.

You see, if two or more EMS workers are left together for any extended period of time, the necessity arises to entertain one another with tales of grueling calls and experiences on the job, each striving only to outdo the previous one. Time after time, we hear co-workers tell outlandish accounts of heroism that include danger, suspense and, of course, humor. The following tips were designed to assist you with this crucial skill and enable you to wax poetic with the best of them.

• The patient's weight plays a critical role in the telling of a war story. Whenever and wherever possible, exaggerate the figures to nearly unbelievable extremes. Just because you mention a figure that exceeds the curb weight of a 747 jumbo jet doesn't mean your co-workers won't believe you. Trust me; it'll work.

• Stairs are extremely important as well. The truly remarkable thing about stairs is that they can

Reprinted with permission from JEMS: Journal of Emergency Medical Services, © 1995; 20(1):125, 127.

exist both inside and outside homes and businesses, allowing several opportunities for embellishment. Include in your story the number of flights, the number of stairs per flight, the ricketiness of the staircase and the size of the stairwell. Combined with the slightly exaggerated weight of your patient, you can create a pretty hair-raising story. Remember one rule of thumb: the sicker and heavier the patient, the higher up he or she will live. Why should a 400-pound patient in acute congestive heart failure live on the ground floor when the ninth will do?

• Believe it or not, equipment failure offers wondrous chances to make yourself into a hero. Listen in awe to the veteran war story teller as he or she recounts the MacGyver-esque modifications made to IV tubing and a catheter during a call; it's truly impressive.

• The worse the weather, the better the story. Heavy rain mixed with hail, sleet, snow or even acid rain makes a great enhancement. Providing the recipient of your war story isn't aware of recent meteorological conditions, you can mention hurricanes, tempests, earthquakes and other incredible acts of God. Why should Dorothy be the only one privileged enough to fly about the countryside in the clutches of a tornado?

• Although we all know that safety is paramount in our industry, personal danger is also a big player in a good war story. Narrowly escaping death to benefit the human race has tremendous and often sobering effects. If you're lucky, you may be able to close the war story session with all your co-workers shaking their heads in awe.

• Keep the number of personnel to a minimum. If possible, try to develop the story so you and your partner are the only providers able to care for the patient. Better still, state that your partner was injured and that you were responsible for the care and handling of both the patient and your partner—while driving the ambulance through a hurricane.

• Empower yourself. This is your story, and like a dream, you have control over the outcome. Give yourself a position of power, some gnarly responsibilities and a lot of obstacles. Speak of the proverbial charter bus that crashes filled with retirees on their way to Las Vegas. Who was the incident commander, primary caregiver, etc.? You!

• Give yourself no room to work with. Mobile homes, trailers, small apartments, economy cars, basements, attics, dog houses, tree houses and that little annoying space between the toilet and shower are all perfect places for a call. You'll get no sympathy if you respond to a mansion; it's got to be small.

• Never make the scene easy to reach. Think about it; we've all been there—the winding, mountainous road to nowhere. Indeed, if you can fashion your story so you were tossed to and fro in the back of a 1976 Dodge ambulance, you'll surely win the hearts of fellow EMS workers.

Remember, these are only guidelines—it is important to develop your own storytelling identity. Think about it; storytelling has been the backbone of many societies, religions and professions. This is not something to be taken lightly. Don't hesitate, don't falter; walk right into that break room or ambulance bay, shake your head, and say, "You'll never guess what happened on this last call. . . ."

Also, don't be shy. Embellish, adjust, alter, modify and transform every detail to your liking. As I mentioned before, this is your story—consider it the verbal equivalent of Play-Doh.

I'll be listening for your tale.

Blueprint for a War Story

The other day, I went on the call from hell. Let me tell you about it. [Partner's name] and I get this call to [location] for a guy complaining of [illness]. Of course, he's on the farthest end of our district and it was [weather condition] outside, and do I even have to tell you the [equipment] wasn't working. I couldn't believe it. Anyway, we finally get to the [location] and find out the guy's apartment is [number] flights up. Of course, the elevator was busted and the patient weighed at least [weight plus 25] pounds.

Just when we get the guy loaded and get a rhythm going down the stairs, [partner's name] hurts his [anatomy], and now I'm taking care of both of them. It was unreal! There were no other [ambulances/firefighters] available, so I'm stuck treating the patient and my partner, not to mention carrying them both down all those stairs. That's when I notice the smoke coming from the building across the street. . . .

WITH APOLOGIES TO ANDY ROONEY

Dexter Hunt, BA, EMT-P

Do you ever wonder why people feel obligated to ask you why the word "ambulance" is spelled backwards on your hood, or why you don't get calls until you start to watch the once-in-a-lifetime TV special?

Do you ever wonder why you always hear "two beers" when you ask someone in an accident how much he had to drink? Seems the reason he crashed was a "little black dog" that ran across the car's path, making it flip. It's obvious our concerns about drunk driving aren't valid. Drinking isn't the problem—it's that dangerous little black dog that causes accidents across the United States. Ever wonder why the dog is always little, black and nowhere to be found when you arrive?

Do you ever wonder why patients lie about how long they've actually had chest pain, the number of pills they took to kill themselves or why they were actually beaten up? The patient tells you he was standing alone on the street corner, minding his own business, when 15 people decided to beat the stuffing out of him. Witnesses note he had questioned the sexual orientation of the mother of everyone in the bar.

Do you ever wonder why administrators really don't have a clue about what's wrong, why fellow employees are capable of denigrating other crew members and why no one ever seems to get a raise except for the absolutely worst employees? In a profession that requires strong individualism, why does management want everyone to be a Pee-wee Herman clone? Do you ever wonder why your coworkers would rather say, "It was an easy call," instead of congratulating you for saving a critical patient?

Have you ever wondered how a nurse can ask you why something wasn't done, while she's standing in a heated, well-lit ED, after you've just spent a half hour of difficult extrication upside down in a blizzard, trying to maintain an airway? Maybe it's a doctor questioning the patency of an endotracheal tube you placed while bullets were flying by.

Do you ever wonder about when rookies will stop spinning circles, chasing their tails at scenes, and why supervisors always assume the worst? How would it be if patients said thank-you for a job well done, instead of complaining about the bill?

Wouldn't it be nice if all of our patients came from clean, fresh-smelling houses and wrapped in cellophane? How would it be if none of our patients ever vomited, urinated or defecated without scheduling it well in advance so we could be off duty?

Do you ever wonder why the burned-out EMTs and paramedics seem to stay with the department longer than the truly gifted? And wouldn't it be great if the truly gifted, compassionate employees could afford to stay?

Wouldn't it be nice if we could take the money we send annually to foreign countries and use it for the health care of the citizens of the United States? Do you ever wonder why some doctors give permission for all of your requests and others deny you the ability to save the patients they've sworn to attempt to heal?

Do you wonder why, in the land of the free, people lock themselves in their houses and apartments so tightly that it makes entry to aid the disabled impossible? Once you get in, do you have to worry about the gun the patient keeps for protection?

Have you ever wondered why there are turf wars when the point of EMS is patient care? Or why we rush trauma scenes to obey the exalted *10-minute limit*, only to have patients lie in the ED for 2 hours and die? Do you ever wonder if the 10-minute limit was ever studied scientifically, or did it come from retrospective findings in one small study?

Do you ever wonder what the point of rapid aeromedical evacuation to a trauma center is when

---

Reprinted with permission from Emergency Medical Services, © 1993; 22(1):74, 72, 73. Edited from the original.

the flight team spends longer at the scene redoing everything that's already been done by the field crew? Do you ever wonder where you find the self-control as you watch someone cut off all of your pressure dressings so he "can see the wound"? Do you ever wonder where egos come from?

Have you ever experienced the excitement of delivering your first baby, only to feel crushed after the supervisor advises you that you didn't dot two i's on the 15 run forms he reviewed? Have you ever wondered why some people have chosen to call patients "clients"? Clients have a choice of care, but most patients don't have the luxury of choice.

For EMS managers: Do you ever wonder if your employees really keep their houses and apartments as they do their quarters—and whether mold is contagious? Do you ever wonder if all of your employees are like little hungry birds, sitting with their mouths open and waiting for the next benefit increase?

Do you ever question your self-control when Person No. 43 in an endless stream of bystanders asks you "if there was an accident" at the scene of the worst multifatality crash you've ever seen? Do you ever wonder why you find yourself calling patients in need "hamsters," "gomers," "skels," "pukes," "scumbags," "fossils," "LOLs," "LOMs," "dirtbags" or worse? Do you ever wonder where cynicism comes from and why you're still reading this article? Do you wonder why, why, why and never get an answer? Do any of these sentences sound familiar? Imagine!

FAMILY FUNCTIONS

Regardless of how many impossible wonders you perform during a shift, that workday will eventually end. We now get to return to those that know us best and still usually welcome our homecoming. Just as at work, we need to become part of a community that will embrace us and enhance our unique strengths and talents. This group with which you share so many mutual interests and feelings was instrumental in shaping your desire to become a health care professional. Hopefully, family will be there to continually remind us of the importance of sharing common bonds and that there is a great life outside of work.

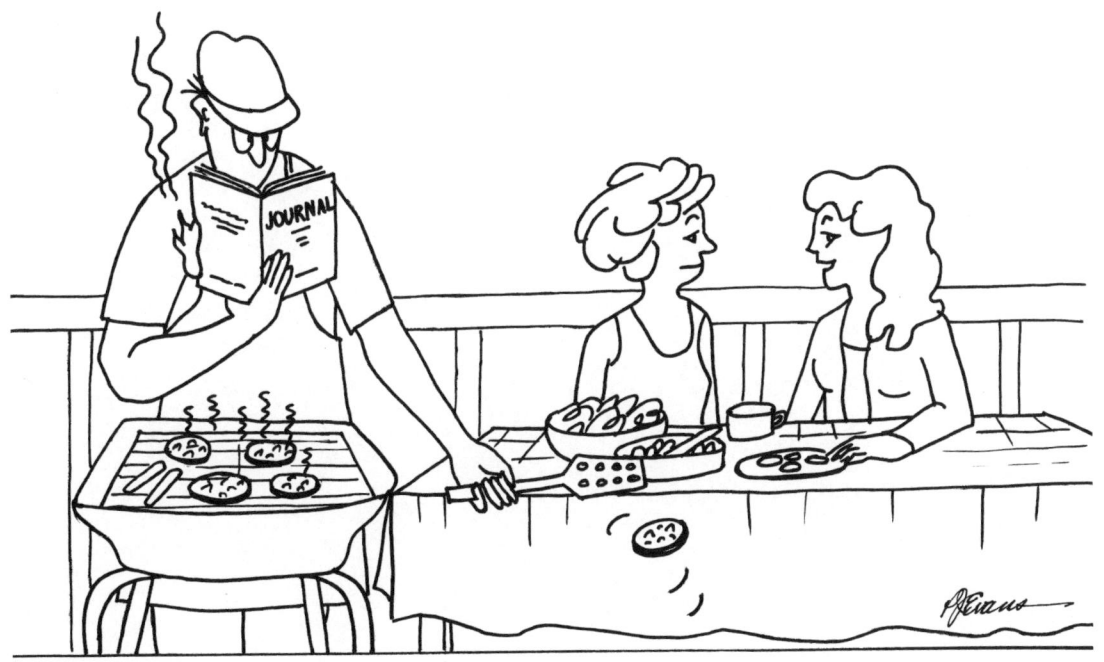

"He claims it's less stressful if he doesn't fall behind with work."

"SO, HERE IT IS SEPTEMBER AGAIN.... LET ME TELL YOU WHAT I DID LAST SUMMER."

Russell L. Malone

Each September the voices of Miss Ashmore, Miss Sedgewick, Miss Sailor, Miss Wallace, Sister Marian Theresa, Miss Miller, Miss Hartman, Miss Love, Miss Bouton, Miss Gerino, Miss Borland, Miss Hendrix, and Miss Purdum come back to me. Each one asks me, "What did you do over your summer vacation?"

I never really had much to say that they'd want to hear. We visited my grandmother, which was pretty boring, especially since she usually spoke French, which I didn't understand. I'd make some extra money by helping my brother deliver the papers. I liked the dime I'd get once a week for helping, because that bought me 10 days of candy and many hours of hassling Mr. Friedlander while I made my daily choice. These events didn't make for an exciting summer. I'd fight with my brother and play ball and go swimming with Denver Yingling and Roy Heyl, but who wants to hear about that? I did some of that every season.

Sometimes we even got in trouble for trying too hard to make our summers sound more interesting. Like the time Roy Heyl reported, in front of our third grade class, that when his family was going to visit his grandfather in the cemetery, his father, a respected businessman in our small community, had leaned out the window to spit out his tobacco and dropped his false teeth on the running board. We all thought that was pretty funny, especially because Mr. Heyl was always very dignified in his three-piece suit. My mother thought it was pretty funny when I told her, and Mrs. Heyl found it funny when Mother told her at Bank Night that Wednesday at the Oaks Theater. But Mr. Heyl did not find it funny when Mrs. Heyl told him, because he didn't chew tobacco or have false teeth.

Of course, sometimes you could get rewarded for what you said. When I was in fifth grade, I reported to Sister Marian Theresa that the highlight of my summer had been going to confession. Sister Marian Theresa smiled beatifically at me, which in itself was very encouraging, since she usually smiled at me only after having cracked me with her ruler.

Sister Marian Theresa was very thorough in her teaching of sin—mortal and venial. She had helped us categorize a good variety of sins under the Seven Deadly Sins and The Ten Commandments. Eating too much pineapple cream pie, I had learned, could fall under the general admonition against GLUTTONY. Studying some of the pictures in *National Geographic* or looking up certain words in the dictionary, I could include under either LUST or ADULTERY. Wanting Denver Yingling's new Tom Mix ring with the secret decoder which would help you understand special messages about Ralston broadcast Mondays through Fridays at 4:00, apparently was classified by God under the sin of ENVY. If I wanted Roy Heyl's secret decoder ring as well, then that was deadly sin #3, AVARICE.

Well, all summer long I had delayed going to confession, but the Saturday before school reopened, I knew I could stall no more. Along with "What did you do over the summer?" would come the ever-popular question, "When did you last go to confession?" So with dread in my heart, fear in my stomach, and a collection of almost 3 months of sins spinning in my memory bank, I waited in the dark confines of the confessional while Father listened to the confession on the other side of his center cubicle. Then I heard the little door to my stall slide open, and I began a recitation that I knew could mean I would spend Saturday afternoon saying rosaries instead of going with Ray Bluestone

Reprinted with permission of the author and ASHA, © 1990; 32(9):96. Edited from the original.

to see the latest Roy Rogers western. Maybe Saturday night, too.

I decided to mix in some of my little sins with my big ones, and say the really bad ones fast. It was a strategy which might cause Father Sanderbeck to miss some of what I said.

"Bless me, Father, for I have sinned. It has been 89 days since my last confession. I have committed these sins. I talked back to my mother and iwaslustful. I fought with my brothers and sisters and icommittedadultry. I told my mother I was studying when I was really reading my new Batman comic book and iwasgluttonous. I talked to Ray Bluestone during mass. I am sorry for these and all the other sins I may have committed."

I was finished. Now, I was going to get it.

"How old are you?" asked Father Sanderbeck.

"Nine."

"Say three Our Fathers and three Hail Marys and a good Act of Contrition."

I couldn't believe it. My strategy had worked! Roy Rogers and Trigger, here I come!

I didn't provide all these details to Sister Marian Theresa, but I told her enough to hold her interest longer than usual. Finally, she interrupted to ask Mary Lou Blinkley about her summer. And, of course, Mary Lou Blinkley, who was the one always charged with taking names of children who talked when Sister left the room, told how she had gone to mass every day and had walked with a stone in her shoe to remind her of the suffering of Christ. But this time, I felt even Mary Lou Blinkley didn't get the same reaction I had from Sister.

What's that, Sister Marian Theresa? It's Mary Lou Blinkley's turn? O.K., talk to you all next September!

STARDOM'S LURE

Ben Dickinson, PharmD student

I learned a valuable lesson from baseball. More specifically, I learned a lesson from Starbrook High's star baseball player, Tommy Morris (not his real name). He hit more home runs and won more awards than anyone else on the team, and I was always jealous of him.

I knew Tommy from summer baseball league. He played shortstop and was Starbrook's superstar. I lived in Crystal Lake, but when I was 12 I started spending the summer in Starbrook with my grandparents. Every summer I played first base on the same team as Tommy. I envied him because he was such a talented—and glorified—player. We had a great summer-league team and were always hard to beat.

The summer before our sophomore year in high school, my mother decided I should live with my grandparents and attend Starbrook High. That summer I spent all my time and energy learning how to swing and throw harder so I could compete with Tommy. *I* wanted to play shortstop and be the town star. The result was ultimate frustration.

Tommy beat me out for shortstop and had an incredible season. He was our fans' favorite player, made the league's Top 10 list almost every week, and was named most valuable player. My season was terrible. I played backup shortstop and batted at the end of the lineup. My throws to first base were wild, and I didn't hit one home run. In fact, I never got on base. I was devastated.

All that hard work and I was having the worst season of my life. I didn't understand it. I had never practiced so hard, and I had never played so poorly. We were well on our way to the state finals when our pitcher was in a car accident and was forced to sit out the rest of the season. Tommy filled in as pitcher, and I was the new starting shortstop. Soon we began to lose. My playing was terrible. We

Reprinted with permission from American Journal of Hospital Pharmacy, © 1994; 51(4):539.

were getting frustrated. The only resemblance to our earlier season was Tommy's outstanding performance. After our last game, I took my frustration out on our first baseman: I told him he should learn how to catch. My temper was flaring and we nearly got into a fight.

Afterwards, Tommy came up to me and said, "You know, at one time you were the best baseball player I knew. Every time you got up to bat, I could count on you to get on base. You were the most accurate and the hardest thrower I knew and you played first base better than anyone else. Now you only hit pop flies for the outfielders to catch, you're a slow and wild thrower, and you're obsessed with playing shortstop. I think *you're* the one who should get it together."

After Tommy left, I just sat there thinking how right he was. I had spent a whole year trying to be somebody else for no reason. I was doing great being myself, but I let jealousy take control. I was so concerned with beating out Tommy as the town star that I lost sight of the facts.

I spent that summer studying techniques of baseball players that I envied, including Tommy. It became clear to me that I was not a power hitter, that I could not throw sidearm, and that I react too slowly to play shortstop. When baseball season came, I tried out for first base. I quit trying to hit a home run every time, and I threw overhand. Our team made it to the state finals. I was named most improved player and was on the Top 10 list a few times. I learned a valuable lesson from that experience that I'll never forget: It is important to recognize the talents and achievements of others so that you can improve upon yourself, but it is even more important to find your own niche in the world.

PUT DOWN THE DUCKIE

Ann F. VanSant, PhD, PT

An article came across my desk regarding knitting in the hospital. The essential message was: knitting in meetings is okay. Scattered through the article are examples of a pediatrician filling "down time" during work at the hospital with knitting. Meetings, grand rounds, continuing education conferences, and other examples of "down time" are provided. And, the author reports being the only student at Harvard who knitted through medical school. The pediatrician speaks of how knitting keeps one focused and brings warm thoughts of the author's child during boring periods of the day. There are also references to carrying heavy medical journals to read but choosing knitting over reading. Speaking of the benefits of revealing our personal interests during our work, this professional likens knitting to bringing in personal mementos to decorate one's office.

But there is a downside to knitting in meetings. As the author notes, some colleagues consider the activity unprofessional. I understand where they are coming from; however, I do not consider knitting unprofessional. I know many professionals who knit, sew, embroider, or crochet. But, I do consider the behavior of focusing attention on knitting rather than participating in professional meetings, conferences, or grand rounds to be rude. This rudeness has nothing to do with professionalism; I would consider the behavior to be rude even among "nonprofessionals."

Where in the world did I get these "outdated" standards of conduct? From two women whom I respect and who taught me how to respect others. One was my mom. She taught me at the same time that she taught me to sew, embroider, and knit, that others could be offended if I chose to knit or embroider, rather than paying attention to them.

The other individual who shaped my beliefs regarding knitting was my former department chair,

Reprinted with permission from Pediatric Physical Therapy, © 1996; 8(4):145. Edited from the original.

Sue Hirt. I was sitting beside her during a district meeting of the Virginia Physical Therapy Association quite a few years ago. A speaker was delivering a talk on Medicare regulations. Probably, the topic would fall into the "boring" category for many, it certainly would have qualified for the pediatrician's definition of "down time." One professional colleague took out her knitting. In a matter of seconds, Sue was kneeling beside the woman quietly and politely requesting that she put the knitting away. "Put down the duckie!"

In a conversation in her office the next day, Sue asked if I was a knitter. "Not a very good one," I replied. Sue had a way of bringing things up gently. She asked for my read on the knitter at the district meeting. I explained my "mother's wit" regarding knitting. She was pleased that this lesson had been learned at home. But, it is possible to knit and listen at the same time, some would argue. Sure it is! But is it possible to knit and demonstrate respect for others simultaneously? I don't think so. Particularly when they are offended by a behavior that signals disinterest to those around them. I genuinely feel that those who choose to bring their hobbies to work and engage in them during meetings or while talking to others are not providing their full measure of attention or respect to their colleagues or their profession. Ernie learned the lesson, so should we: "Put down the duckie if you want to play the saxophone."

THE MALE MIDLIFE CRISIS

Theodore E. Keats, MD

As chairman of a large radiology department, one must wear many hats. One of those that I have assumed without prior training is that of mentor, counselor, and armchair psychiatrist to my staff. When you gather this many people together in an organization and you are responsible for their welfare, it is inevitable that their problems become a part of your life as well. Out of this cornucopia, there is one problem that is most intriguing that I would like to discuss here: namely, the male midlife crisis. This entity is well-documented in the psychology literature and represents one of the normal "passages" of the male. It strikes in midlife, between 45 and 55 years of age, when the subject has climbed most of his mountains and can reflect on his life and accomplishments. This may be a comforting and reassuring experience or it may incite panic, as our subject becomes aware of his own mortality and the fact that his life is more than half over. If there are dreams that remain unfulfilled, they now become terrifyingly important and there is a need for urgency of action. In my experience, the subject usually takes one of the following courses of action:

1. Gets a divorce. A new wife often restores his self-esteem and lends a new air of accomplishment. He is still in the running.

2. Takes a mistress. This produces many of the rewards of option 1 but in a more dangerous fashion.

3. Takes a new job. This may provide him with more money, a change of scene, new colleagues, and new challenges. Wise and lasting decisions are not always a product of this choice.

4. Gets a new red sports car. This is a dramatic statement and usually the least damaging in the long term.

It is important to know that the syndrome under discussion has a limited life expectancy and will pass in time. The role of the mentor in dealing with the syndrome is to urge patience and the avoidance of radical alterations in life style until the wave of urgency for action has passed. Such counseling is not always successful and nature must take its course. Personally, I push the red sports car whenever possible.

Reprinted with permission from Applied Radiology, © 1991; 20(6):15.

THE VIEW ASKEW

Pat Vietenthal, RN

Woe to be the Kid of Nurse! Just ask my son. He's a rather verbal 10 year old who claims to be highly insulted that I never take his complaints of illness or injury seriously. Sound familiar? It infuriates him that each ache or pain is met with the gentle response, "Suck it up kid! I'm an ED nurse. I know what 'hurt' REALLY looks like!" (Besides, aren't 10 year olds always either ill, injured, verbal, or highly insulted?)

These were, in fact, my very words to him when he fell off of his skateboard and landed on his left arm a while ago. Four days later, the EMT father of my son's playmate was kind enough to bring my son to me at work after noticing that he was not using his left arm at all. The EMT thought I would want to know this right away. He also thought that whatever happened was probably *his* kid's fault and was interrogating him intensely. X-rays, of course, revealed that my son's left elbow was fractured in two places. Now I admit, I was perfectly willing to let the playmate take the rap, but my son, AKA The Informer (who is a great deal like his father), arose piously from his seat, and announced within earshot of at least 3 neighboring states that his elbow had actually *been this way for 4 days*, and that his mother, *The ED Nurse* had known about it the whole time!

My colleagues then began asking my son if I had, in fact, PUSHED him off his skateboard, Human Resources did a repeat background check (and I swear I heard someone whisper Child Protective Services), and the heroic EMT stopped allowing his kid, who no longer speaks to me, to come over to our house. But since that silly little incident, I've noticed that my son has become very wise. He obviously began to study what I do for a living, because he has learned how to get attention. In fact, he's gotten so good at it that he has actually complained of chest pain (with shortness of breath yet!) because he knows that it's triaged "Emergent"! Not when I was around mind you, but needless to say this terrified his father on more than one occasion, causing panicky phone calls to me at work . . . (but why should he believe my attempts at reassurance? After all, I missed the boy's elbow fracture . . .!) Not to mention what I did to his poor grandmother who still doesn't believe that I even graduated from high school, let alone two nursing schools! (Just because I played a little hooky in the 60's for Gosh sakes!) She's ready to mortgage her home to bribe Christiaan Barnard out of retirement for a Cardiac Consultation! Anyway, I gave my son a 6.425 for Originality, but told him he'd have to work on "cyanosis" before I was having any of it. But it does seem to be different for the Kids of Nurses, doesn't it? They do seem to have to "push the buttons" a bit harder than most kids. The RN who is the school nurse at my son's primary school is a friend of mine, and she tells me she can spot the Kid of a Nurse instantly.

She says they always know how to act really sick, rarely are really sick, and use phrases like "nuchal rigidity"! Yeah, it can be rough to be a nurse's kid, but it sure isn't all bad. OK, so we miss an elbow or two every once in a while, but nurses' kids usually have "up to date" immunizations, and they're more likely to wear helmets, and seatbelts (and elbow pads which he had but didn't put on!) They're usually the first kids to learn their addresses and phone numbers, and they know that 911 is for emergencies long before they ever see it on TV! They know things like Stop, Drop and Roll, and many of them know how to do CPR at a very early age. My son will even follow his 2-year-old cousin around removing what he refers to as "Potential Airway Obstructions" from her path. Being the Kid of a Nurse is actually a pretty big deal when you stop and think about it. Just ask my 10 year old and he'll tell you. In fact, he'll tell you *anything* you want to know. Just *please* don't ask him about the change jar in his room labeled Future Therapy Fund. . . .

Reprinted with permission from Revolution: The Journal of Nurse Empowerment, © 1997; 7(1):59.

LESSONS IN DEPENDENCY:

Advice from A Failure
Bob Demers, BS, RRT

Some people maintain that it is inappropriate to espouse a particular virtue unless the one doing so is completely virtuous. This school of thought holds that parents should abstain from telling their children not to lie if they themselves indulge in "little white lies."

I think someone is often better equipped to advise others about snares and pitfalls after having been ensnared oneself.

Years ago, I needed to learn some lessons about dependence and independence. In the process of learning those lessons, and partially because I was such a slow learner, my marriage failed. To my surprise, however, I discovered that failure can be a uniquely effective means of education. I would like to relate some of these hard-learned lessons. Just think of it as advice from a failure.

It took me longer than most to shed my air of independence after I got married. All too frequently, I would make a commitment or formulate plans without first consulting my patient and often frustrated spouse. On more than one occasion, I even had the audacity to invite people over for dinner, consulting my wife only after the fact! Obviously, it is not only inconvenient, but downright damaging when one member of a team ignores the other member(s) and acts as a free agent. The addition of new members to the team (such as children) compounds the problem exponentially.

After (too) many moons, I finally divested myself of the completely independent mind-set that was more appropriate for a single bachelor than for a husband and father. Unfortunately, though, I unconsciously adopted a mentality that was fully as inappropriate and destructive: one of total dependence. Without realizing it at the time, I utterly relinquished my independence. In the process, whatever vestiges of autonomy I had had were abandoned.

It is easy to see why utter dependence of this type is so destructive; it puts the other person under incredible pressure to shoulder the burdens of coping virtually single-handedly with every situation that presents itself. Furthermore, whatever strengths and talents the depender might have originally had are nullified as that person strives to become little more than a clone of his counterpart.

I learned a valuable lesson from this experience: there is a third alternative to complete independence or complete dependence. This alternative consists of a healthy and growth-inducing interdependence. When the members of a team are interdependent, the talents, strengths, and insights of each person are pooled to the mutual benefit of each. In addition, the faults or failings of individual team members can be minimized by the assumption of roles where those particular shortcomings become irrelevant. And, as so frequently observed in the context of the athletic team, an outstanding level of performance by one team member can serve as a powerful potentiator of improved performance by each and every member of that team.

No doubt, you're wondering why I'm waxing philosophic like this and not in a column to "Dear Abby." Well, the lessons I learned about independence, dependence, and interdependence have carried over into my professional life. A letter that I received in response to an editorial about medical direction succeeded in crystallizing some of the thoughts written here. The writer of that letter disapproved of my allegiance to the notion of maintaining respiratory therapists' ties with physicians. While we all would like to condemn the picture of the therapist who is slavishly deferential to physicians, wholly lacking any professional identity, fawning, servile, and obsequious, we should be careful about seeking completely independent practice for respiratory care practitioners.

Reprinted with permission from AARC Times, © 1992; 16(10):6–7. Edited from the original.

The *interdependent* therapist is a role model we would do well to emulate. Interdependent therapists are the best caregivers they can be, exercising their knowledge and talent within the context of the team approach. In this environment, each caregiver contributes to the welfare of the patient and to the viability of the team that administers care.

Individual members' assertion of their professionalism reinforces—not undermines—the contributions of the team. And, because individual team members need not be concerned about jockeying for position within a prevailing "pecking order," no one is prompted to be envious or jealous of other members' respective roles.

OF CATS, DOGS, AND DRUG INTERACTIONS

Philip D. Hansten, PharmD

The neighbors brought home an Airedale, and our female half-Siamese was not pleased. Now, whenever she went out the front door she had to make a dash for the blackberries to escape his murderous assault. Stealth was not his forte, so she always heard him coming. But, we began to feel guilty for having her front claws removed (especially since we had sensibly waited until she had ruined the couch). After several months of these daily attacks, the neighbor installed an "invisible fence." This consisted of a wire buried around the perimeter of his yard, marked with flags, and a small gray box on the dog's neck. When the dog got within about 2 meters of the wire the box buzzed his neck; if he crossed the wire it gave him a painful electric shock. It took our cat about a week to figure out that, somehow, mysteriously, the dog could not venture beyond those little white flags. She then began an activity that can only be termed perverse—she began to taunt the dog daily. Miss Nonchalant, sitting just outside the white flags, licking herself, and occasionally strolling back and forth. The dog, meanwhile, is having apoplexy on the other side, barking and jumping, and running back and forth. Every now and then our neighbor would inform us that our cat was "torturing their dog again." I am sure that during this time the cat told all of her cat friends, "Well, in my clinical experience it's perfectly safe; just be sure not to go past the white flags." Then after several months of this antisocial behavior, a strange thing happened. We never found out whether the batteries in the dog's collar went dead, or perhaps he just said to himself, "Okay, that's it! I don't care if they electrocute me—I'm going to GET that cat!" In any case, he broke free one day, and our cat lost faith in judgments based solely on clinical experience. She never taunted him again. Apparently, the uncertainty was too much for her.

For many drug interactions, our understanding of why one person manifests an adverse outcome and the next person does not is only marginally better than our cat's understanding of batteries and electricity.

So, because drug interactions can be unpredictable, should we always avoid giving interacting drug combinations? Of course not. After considering the specific situation we may decide that the benefit of using an interacting combination is greater than the risk of an adverse outcome. But to be intellectually honest, we must acknowledge that such judgments are usually based on woefully inadequate data. Such decisions are, in large part, educated guesses. But, that is better than an *uneducated* guess (or no guess at all). Moreover, uncertainty is not all

© 1995 by Lippincott/Raven Publishers. Reprinted with permission from *Hospital Pharmacy*, 1995 edition. St. Louis, MO: Facts and Comparisons, a Wolters Kluwer Company.

bad. In his biography of physicist Richard Feynman, author James Gleick pointed out that Feynman embraced uncertainty. Feynman celebrated the fact that, although we know that we can never be more than provisionally right on any given topic, we are able to act nevertheless. The irony is that one of the most brilliant physicists of all time readily embraced and acknowledged uncertainty in a "hard" field such as physics, while certitude and dogmatism are so prevalent in the "softer" fields of pharmacy and medicine. (Although Feynman embraced uncertainty in physics, he didn't *embrace all* uncertainty; when he remarried in his early 40s, his new wife found five identical pairs of shoes in his closet!)

What are the practical lessons of uncertainty in handling drug interactions? I think there are at least three: (1) clinical decisions are likely to be better if one honestly faces the limitations of the available data; (2) an up-front admission that predicting the outcome of drug interactions is an inexact science helps to preserve your credibility if your prediction is off the mark; and (3) greater civility might be evident in disputes among clinicians over the importance of drug interactions. So, like Richard Feynman, we should embrace rather than eschew, uncertainty. It makes life more interesting, and without it, the clinical judgment of the pharmacist would become a vestigial function.

THANKSGIVING?

Mary Grayson

Thanksgiving is not one of my favorite holidays. This was always the day my parents invited to dinner every sourpuss relative, quarrelsome neighbor, and self-righteous jerk we knew. None of us could stand them, but for whatever reason, my parents felt a sense of obligation to include them in a social event at least once a year. So they ganged them all together in one excruciating afternoon every Thanksgiving. It was sort of like having all your teeth pulled at once.

The guests were a grumpy bunch who invariably thought children should be seen and not heard and that dogs should never be allowed in the house because they are dirty and spread germs. And cats. Well, everybody knows that cats carry the bubonic plague!

Whenever my two sisters and I would groan about the upcoming day of "thanksgiving" to be spent with the usual bunch of crab apples, my mother would say: "Well, so-and-so hasn't had an easy life." Or, "Ya know, living by yourself for a long time tends to make people a little odd." I'll say. Apparently, it also makes some people mean and stingy. Well, Mom, there was a good reason why most of those people ended up living by themselves. No one could stand being around them. And some people with arduous lives actually have pleasant dispositions.

Years later, my sister Patsy and I were having dinner in a restaurant, sitting next to a group of particularly unpleasant people. They complained about everything and drove the young waitress to the brink of tears. Patsy commented that they must all have had "one heck of a hard life," and that it was a good thing Dad wasn't there "because he would have invited them all to our house for Thanksgiving dinner." She was only half kidding.

When the dreaded day came, we kids were not only not heard, but we tried to be seen as little as possible, so as to avoid lectures about how worthless and disrespectful "young people are today."

No one had the heart to put old Fido, our mongrel bird dog, out in the cold, damp autumn air for the afternoon. So Fido would retreat—germs and all—to the deepest, darkest corner of the big walk-in

Reprinted from *Hospitals & Health Networks*, Vol. 71, No. 22, by permission, November 20, 1997. Copyright 1997, by Health Forum, Inc.

closet and stay there until it was safe to come out. Occasionally, Fido would give out a low, sad moan that we could all relate to, but would deny hearing when our grumpy guests demanded, "What was that?"

As for the cats—well, they acted like cats. Confounded by their sudden exclusion, they thought we had just made some horrible mistake and didn't really intend to lock them out of the house. They tried to bring this "oversight" to our attention by going from windowsill to windowsill and parading back and forth while howling at the top of their lungs. "Look at those dirty, plague-carrying cats," our guests would say.

All in all, though, there were still things to be thankful for. For one, most of the guests fell asleep after eating too much for dinner, and they went home early because being with other people was too annoying. Fido would then come out and the cats would leap in.

Sometimes, we in health care get a little grumpy. We think we live hard lives, and we focus on all the bad things. But we are at the center of one of the most interesting and important periods in health care. Stop and enjoy the significance of your job and good work. Or you'll end up living alone. And since my father is no longer alive, there will be no one to invite you over for turkey.

THE FOLLY OF FAMILY VACATIONS

Dave Barry

Parents, school is almost out, which means it's time to make those summer vacation plans, load up the family car and take off, quickly, before the kids get home.

I am of course joshing. You should take the kids; there's nothing quite like putting the whole family into the car and hitting the open road, leaving your worries behind, driving mile after carefree mile, sometimes getting as many as three carefree miles before everybody in the car hates everybody else and gunfire breaks out in the back seat.

Yes, medical emergencies can occur on even the best-planned family trip. That's why, before you set out, you should familiarize yourself with the:

OFFICIAL GOVERNMENT CLASSIFICATIONS OF BAD MEDICAL THINGS THAT COULD HAPPEN ON YOUR VACATION

I refer here to the International Classification of Diseases (ICD), which is the system used to report medical problems to US government agencies.

Alert reader Denise Martin sent me a copy of the ICD, which classifies every conceivable kind of medical problem, including the following, which I am not making up:

E845—Accident in spacecraft
E912—Bean in nose
E966—Beheaded by guillotine
E906.8—Butted by animal
E842—Glider fire
E915—Hairball
E908—Injured by cloudburst
E912—Marble in nose
E906.8—Pecked by bird
E844—Sucked into jet aircraft

Do not let this list alarm you. Statistics show that, on any given vacation trip, your family is likely to experience no more than four or five of these emergencies—even fewer, if you exercise strict parental discipline ("Jason, you let your brother out of that guillotine RIGHT NOW, or we are NOT stopping at the Tastee Freeze").

© Tribune Media Services, Inc. All Rights Reserved. Reprinted with permission.

Speaking of sharp objects, you'll want to be especially careful if your vacation destination includes a rain forest. I say this because of an alarming experience I had last summer when the Barry family held a reunion on the Olympic Peninsula in Washington. One afternoon a bunch of us Barrys packed some healthy trail provisions in the form of a large box of Cheez-Its and drove to the Quinault Rain Forest, which is one of those nature preserves where they put up lots of informational signs with drawings of specific wildlife items that you never see anywhere except on the signs.

For example, if the sign says that the area is the natural habitat of the River Otter, you can be sure that there will be no River Otters within miles of it. The River Otters, who can read at a sixth-grade level, will all be deliberately hanging around the sign for some OTHER animal, such as the Toe-Sucking Bigtail Bat, which meanwhile will be hanging around yet ANOTHER animal's sign. This pattern continues throughout the animal kingdom, forming what zoologists call the Great Chain of Totally Incorrect Nature Signs.

Anyway, we went to the Quinault Rain Forest to expose the younger generation of Barrys to nature and teach them to appreciate the vital ecological importance of our dwindling rain forests, without which the world would soon run completely out of mildew. The first thing we saw, on arriving in the rain forest parking lot, was a bulletin board with a recently tacked-up notice that said, I swear:

ATTENTION!! THIS PERSON IS KNOWN TO BE IN THIS AREA.

(This was followed by the person's name and physical description, then:)

LAST SEEN WEARING EARRINGS, A TATTOO (ON SHOULDER), CAMOUFLAGED PANTS (MILITARY TYPE), AND A VEST. CARRYING A MACHETE.

THIS PERSON HAS ASSAULTED A GOVERNMENT EMPLOYEE AND IS CONSIDERED DANGEROUS.

As you can imagine, this notice put something of a damper on our rain forest experience. It's difficult to fully appreciate the habitat of the Northern Flying Squirrel when you are expected at any moment to encounter the Camouflaged Machete Loon.

Nevertheless we followed the little nature trail and read all the informational signs, which appeared to have been written by graduates of Extremely Creative Writing 101. For example, at one point my brother Sam and I were munching Cheez-Its and reading a sign that said, quote:

> "Lean your head back; peer into the forest canopy. Search for the subtle activity and listen as the gentle breezes muffle the sounds of life above."

"Are you gonna do that?" I asked Sam. "I'd be afraid that a squirrel would go to the bathroom on my face," he replied. For some reason, I feel compelled to point out here that Sam is a Presbyterian minister.

Anyway, we got out of the rain forest without any mishaps, and I'm sure that by now the machete person has been captured by the authorities or eaten by otters. So you and your family probably have nothing to worry about this summer; just relax, have fun, and enjoy a totally carefree vacation, wherever you roam, from Sea to Shining Sea. Speaking of which, E906.3 is the ICD code for shark bite.

THE OT SPOUSE

J. W. Yeager

I've often wondered why the spouses of occupational therapists haven't received the national recognition they rightly deserve.

It's a thankless job, I assure you. After all, we seem to be the ones the therapists practice the therapy on before putting it into use.

In the three years that my wife has been completing her education, I've had cock-up splints made for my hands, been subjected to behavior modification (didn't work), had my range of motion tested numerous times, and, while helping her study, have inadvertently memorized all the nerves in the body.

My study was taken over by a massive craft project. I was sent on an expedition looking for old bottles to dismember, and even had my Sunday afternoon naps interrupted by a noisy wood project.

I am now equipped to sit at social functions and chit-chat fluently about ADL or Rohlfing, and can explain what Occupational Therapy is in 25 words or less.

I've been through the school-time jitters, the affiliation jitters, the graduation jitters, and the registration ("I'll never pass it!") exam jitters.

Our closets are filled with enough macrame supplies to make a belt for every man, woman, and child in the United States. I've purchased enough devices for rug hooking, leather work, beading, and tools to find it difficult to believe that our country has been through an economic crisis.

I've learned that nothing should be thrown away because somewhere, someday, an occupational therapist can make something out of it.

By the way, is there a clinic somewhere that would be interested in purchasing 15,000 yards of jute? How about 500 empty bottles, or 3,000 egg cartons?

From American Journal of Occupational Therapy; 30(7):453. Copyright 1976 by the American Occupational Therapy Association, Inc. Reprinted with permission.

BOOK BIBLIOGRAPHY

Barron, James W. (ed): Humor and Psyche: Psychoanalytic Perspectives. Hillsdale, NJ, Analytic Press, 1999.

Bennett, Howard J: The Best of Medical Humor: A Collection of Articles, Essays, Poetry, and Letters Published in the Medical Literature, 2nd edition. Philadelphia, Hanley & Belfus, 1997.

Bosker, Gideon: Medicine is the Best Laughter: A Second Dose. St. Louis, Mosby, 1998.

Davies, Christie: Jokes and their Relation to Society. Berlin, Mouton de Gruyter, 1998.

Davis, Murray S: What's So Funny? The Comic Conception of Culture and Society. Chicago, University of Chicago Press, 1993.

DuPre, Athena. Humor and the Healing Arts: A Multimethod Analysis of Humor Use in Health Care. Mahwah, NJ, Lawrence Erlbaum Associates, 1998.

Harvey, Linda C: Humor for Healing: A Therapeutic Approach. San Antonio, Therapy Skill Builders, 1998.

Jackson, MM: The comedy of management, pp 339–351. In LM Simms, SA Price, NE Ervin (eds): The Professional Practice of Nursing Administration. New York, John Wiley & Sons, 1985.

Kenefick, Colleen and Young, Amy Y: The Best of Nursing Humor: A Collection of Articles, Essays, and Poetry Published in the Nursing Literature, Volume 2. Philadelphia, Hanley & Belfus, Inc., 1999.

Kenefick, Colleen and Young, Amy Y: The Best of Nursing Humor: A Collection of Articles, Essays, and Poetry Published in the Nursing Literature. Philadelphia, Hanley & Belfus, Inc., 1993.

London, Fran: Never a dull moment, pp 109–143. In London F: No Time to Teach? A Nurse's Guide to Patient and Family Education. Philadelphia, Lippincott, 1999.

Peterson, KE: The use of humor in AIDS prevention, in the treatment of HIV-positive persons, and in the remediation of caregiver burnout, pp 37–57. In MR Seligson, KE Peterson (eds): Aids Prevention and Treatment: Hope, Humor and Healing. New York, Hemisphere, 1992.

Rabin, Bruce S: Stress, Immune Function, and Health: The Connection. New York, Wiley-Liss, 1999.

Slack, Jonathan MW: Egg and Ego: An Almost True Story of Life in the Biology Lab. New York, Springer, 1998.

JOURNAL BIBLIOGRAPHY

Admonitions

Which humour for doctors? Lancet 1998 Jan 3; 351(9095): 1.

Abdulla S: Heard the one about having a laugh? London Financial Times 1999 Mar 11:15.

Benatar D: Prejudice in jest: When racial and gender humor harms. Public Affairs Quarterly 1999 Apr; 13(2):191–203.

Chapman T: Cleaning up bad behavior in the OR. Surgical Technologist 1999 Jan; 31(1):22–25.

Gabriel Y: An introduction to the social psychology of insults in organizations. Human Relations 1998 Nov; 51(11):1329–1354.

Gaut B: Just joking: The ethics and aesthetics of humor. Philosophy and Literature 1998 Apr; 22(1):51–68.

McCaffery M: Is laughter the best medicine? American Journal of Nursing 1998 Dec; 98(12):12.

Mango-Hurdman C, Richman J: A note on ethnicity in humor and art therapy. Art Therapy 1994; 11(3):214–215.

Olschewski G: Your idea of humor may not be the same as your patients'. RN 1998 Oct; 61(10):10.

Sweeney K: Patch Adams the movie: Laughter makes for bad medicine. Trustee 1999 Apr; 52(4):22–23.

Wallace S: Healing with humor: Comic relief and caveats. Alternative & Complementary Therapies 1999 Dec; 5(6):390.

Departmental Uses

Creativity catches on with ED staff. Healthcare Benchmarks 1999 Feb; 6(2):19–20.

Humor and histology: A healthy mix. Canadian Journal of Medical Technology 52(4):256–257.

Asa R: Thrill of victory lights team spirit in materials management olympics. Materials Management in Health Care 1996 Jul; 5(7):20.

Ashworth P: Humour—A critical faculty in critical care nursing? Intensive & Critical Care Nursing 1999 Oct; 15(5):245.

Barnes II: Toward a caring dementia unit. Canadian Nursing Home 1997 Mar; 8(1):15–16, 18–21.

Basmajian JV: The elixir of laughter in rehabilitation. Archives of Physical Medicine and Rehabilitation 1998 Dec; 79(12):1597.

Beck CT: Humor in nursing practice: A phenomenological study. International Journal of Nursing Studies 1997 Oct; 34(5): 346–352.

Kuska B: A tale of too witty? Using whimsy to name fringe genes. Journal of the National Cancer Institute 1997 Oct 1; 89(19):1396–1397.

Mango CR, Richman J: Humor and art therapy. American Journal of Art Therapy 1990 May; 28(4):111–114.

Mattera MD: Nursing lite. RN 1998 Jul; 61(7):7.

Miller LD: Humor as a projective technique in occupational therapy. American Journal of Occupational Therapy 1970 Apr; 24(3):201–204.

Nelson DS: Humor in the pediatric emergency department: A 20-year retrospective. Pediatrics 1992 Jun; 89(6):1089–1090.

Parrish MM, Quinn P: Laughing your way to peace of mind: How a little humor helps caregivers survive. Clinical Social Work Journal 1999 Sum; 27(2):203–211.

Peace BL: President's message. Journal of the American Medical Record Association 1990 Sep; 61(9):29–30.

Thornton J, White A: Heideggerian investigation into the lived experience of humour by nurses in an intensive care unit. Intensive & Critical Care Nursing 1999 Oct; 15(5):266–278.

Tierney WM: Laughter and balance: A letter to a junior resident. Journal of General Internal Medicine 1998 Apr; 13(4): 271–272.

Tuinstra SEB: You had to be there: True stories of humor in the OR. Seminars in Perioperative Nursing 1999 Apr; 8(2):88–94.

Zundel KM: The effects of residency on the mental health of a hospital librarian. Bulletin of the Medical Library Association 1989 Oct; 77(4):384–386.

Education

Bust stress with humor, yoga inservices. Homecare Education Management 1998 Dec; 3(12):186–187.

Here are stress-relief tips for your next inservice: three educators offer their ideas. Homecare Education Management 1998 Dec; 3(12):187–188.

Beitz JM: Keeping them in stitches: Humor in perioperative education. Seminars in Perioperative Nursing 1999 Apr; 8(2):71–79.

Berk RA, Nanda JP: Effects of jocular instructional methods on attitudes, anxiety, and achievement in statistics courses. Humor 1998; 11(4):383–409.

Bizzaro MP, Gardner A, Putz M: Mission nutrition. Journal of Nutrition Education 1995 May/Jun; 27(3):157–158.

Brown AP: Using games to teach. Journal of Emergency Nursing 1999 Oct; 25(5):415–416.

Burke S: Childbirth classroom: Using humor when teaching. Childbirth Instructor Magazine 1998 Mar/Apr; 8(2):46–47.

Ducrot J, Mastromarino JC: Iseo and the ostomates. World Council of Enterostomal Therapists Journal 1994 Apr/Jun; 14(2):22–24.

Fishman PB: Teaching nutrition with magic. Journal of the American Dietetic Association 1980 Nov; 77(5):580–582.

Flournoy E, Turner G, Combs D: Critical care nurses read the writing on the wall. Nursing Management 2000 Feb; 31(2):46.

Freeman L: Clowning around for a good cause. Emergency Medical Services 1994 Mar; 23(3):38.

Grady K, Glazer G: Humor in prenatal education: From egg to eggplant. Journal of Perinatal Education 1994; 3(3):15–21.

Graham K: Straight talk and humour: Adolescent sexual issues. Lamp 1997 Oct; 54(9):16.

Hansen S: Adding pizazz to childbirth education. International Journal of Childbirth Education 1993 Mar; 8(1):11–12.

Heckerson EW: The teacher has done his homework . . . but are we having fun yet? Emergency Medical Services 1996 Oct; 25(10):41–42, 72.

Henderson T, Cumming B: An innovative teaching strategy for staff development departments: Olga and Bertha to the rescue. Journal of Nursing Staff Development 1997 Jul/Aug; 13(4):183–188, 235.

Henneman AC: Teaching nutrition to nursing students: Let's have a party! Journal of the American Dietetic Association 1978 Nov; 73(5):546.

Huntsucker CR: Fun and games with asthma management. RT: The Journal for Respiratory Care Practitioners 1992 Apr/May; 5(3):91–92.

Loring CF: Do nurses really eat their young? AWHONN Lifelines 1999 Feb/Mar; 3(1):47–50.

McMorris RF, Boothroyd RA, Pietrangelo DJ: Humor in educational testing: A review and discussion. Applied Measurement in Education 1997; 10(3):269–297.

Nahas VL: Humour: A phenomenological study within the context of clinical education. Nurse Education Today 1998 Nov; 18(8):663–672.

Perlini AH, Nenonen RG, Lind DL: Effects of humor on test anxiety and performance. Psychological Reports 1999 Jun; 84(3 Pt 2):1203–1213.

Safford F: Humor as an aid in gerontological education. Gerontology & Geriatrics Education 1991; 11(3):27–37.

Shultz K, Germeroth D: Should we laugh or should we cry? John Callahan's humor as a tool to change societal attitudes toward disability. Howard Journal of Communications 1998 Jul/Sep; 9(3):229–244.

Tow PK, Tonelson S: An exercise on enacting proverbs in health education. Journal of Health Education 1994 Jul/Aug; 25(4):247–248.

Williams BL, Hubbard B: Teaching theory through cartoons. Journal of Health Education 1994 May/Jun; 25(3):179–180.

Ziegler JB: Humour in medical teaching. Medical Journal of Australia 1999 Dec 6; 171(11–12):579–580.

Zimmerman M, Harold R: Taking the labor out of childbirth education classes. International Journal of Childbirth Education 1991 Aug; 6(3):13–14.

Healing Power of Humor

Adams P: Fun and the joy of service. Townsend Letter for Doctors and Patients 1998 Jul; 180:89–90.

Chowka PB: Bernie Siegel, M.D.: Turning modern medicine upside down. Nutrition Science News 1997 Mar; 2(3):110–112.

Dayton L: Healing with humor. Clowns on call bring hugs and happiness. Michigan Health & Hospitals 1997 Sep/Oct; 33(5):16.

Ferguson ER: Can laughter every day keep the doctor away? Alternative Medicine 2000 Jan; 33:70.

Foltz-Gray D: Make 'em laugh. Humor programs can help residents heal—Seriously. Contemporary Longterm Care 1998 Sep; 21(9):44–46, 48, 50.

Hammerschlag C: Wisdom and health in spirit, mind, and body. Caring 1999 Oct; 18(10):14–16, 18–19.

Rader R: Keeping them in stitches—How humor helps healing happen. Exceptional Parent 1999 Jun; 29(6):47–58, 60.

Sherman KM: Healing with humor. Seminars in Perioperative Nursing 1998 Apr; 7(2):128–137.

Smith N: Is laughter the best medicine? American Journal of Nursing 1998 Dec; 98(12):12, 14.

Ward SL: Caring and healing in the 21st century. MCN 1998 Jul/Aug 1998; 23(4):210–215.

Improving Your Sense of Humor

Barros A: Is the sky really falling? MLO 1986 Aug; 18(8):21.

Brown L: Laughter: The best medicine. Canadian Journal of Medical Radiation Technology 1991 Aug; 22(3):127–129.

Campbell AJ: Using humor in medical practice. Missouri Medicine 1997 Oct; 94(10):603.

Culberson RP: Humor at work: Could this keep staff happy? Caring 2000 Apr; 19(4):44–45.

Dina G: How do we develop humor? The Delta Kappa Gamma Bulletin 1999 Spr; 65(3):37.

Fonnesbeck BG: Are you kidding? If you're not, maybe you should think about using a lighter touch with your patients. Nursing 1998 Mar; 28(3):64.

Francis L, Monahan K, Berger C: A laughing matter? The uses of humor in medical interactions. Motivation and Emotion 1999 Jun; 23(2):155–174.

Grensing-Pophal L: Getting your dose of laughter. Nursing 1999 Feb; 29(2):56.

Hague DA: Balancing the demands in your life through humor. Ohio Nurses Review 1994 Jan/Feb; 69(1):9–11, 13.

Harmon S: How to become changehardy. Medical Laboratory Observer 1993 Aug; 25(8):41–45, 48.

Insel PM: Humor can lighten your load! Healthline 1996 Sep; 15(9):9.

London A: HumoRoundup! Laughter Prescription 1996 Oct; 8(5):1, 3.

McGarey W: Joy for long life, doctors advise. Pathways to Health 1995 Jun; 4(1):1, 4.

McGhee P: Laughter & health: Humor helps prevent illness, humor helps heal illness: Simple secrets of a great sense of humor. Bottom Line/Health 1998 Apr; 12(4):7–9.

McMillan L. The new miracle drug: Laughter! Vibrant Life 1996 Sep/Oct; 12(5):4–5.

Nordberg M: Laughing with Loretta. Emergency Medical Services 1996 Jan; 25(1):27.

Pfifferling J, Gilley K: Putting "life" back into your professional life. Family Practice Management 1999 Jun; 6(6):36–42, 57–58.

Pilla LM: Lightening up. Nursing 1998 Jun; 28(6):10.

Rogalin E: The grin doctors: It's ironic, but humor has taken a turn for the serious. Body Mind Spirit 1997 Oct; 16(4):33–37.

Selzman LJ: Let it go: 5 ways to alleviate everyday anxiety. American Health 1999 Jan; 18(1):62–65.

Strickland D: Overcome terminal seriousness: Let go, laugh, and lighten up! Seminars in Perioperative Nursing 1999 Apr; 8(2):53–59.

Terry AA: Taking life too seriously? Tips on how to lighten up. Conscious Choice 1997 Jun; 10(3):48–49.

Unland MK, Kleiner BH: How to enhance one's sense of humor. American Journal of Management Development 1995; 1(4): 9–14.

Witkin SL: Taking humor seriously. Social Work 1999 Mar; 44(2):101–104.

Wooten P: You've got to be kidding! Humor skills for surviving managed care. Dermatology Nursing 1997 Dec; 9(6):423–429.

Management

Hoping to influence patient satisfaction levels, Integris goes for laughs. The funniest hospital in Oklahoma. Profiles in Healthcare Marketing 1997 Jan/Feb; 13(1):11–14

Barbour G: Want to be a successful manager? Now that's a laughing matter! Public Management 1998 Jul; 80(7):6–9.

Boe GP: How to deal with stress in the laboratory. Medical Laboratory Observer 1981 Apr; 13(4):149–154.

Davidhizar R, Shearer R: Humor: Don't manage people without it. Radiologic Technology 1997 Sep/Oct; 69(1):83–87.

Davis KG: Communication skills: Physician, laugh at thyself. Family Practice Management 1998 Sep; 5(8):72, 75.

Grahl C: Singing the managed care blues. Behavioral Health Management 1998 Sep: 37.

Hatch MJ: Irony and the social construction of contradiction in the humor of a management team. Organization Science 1997 May/Jun; 8(3):275–288.

Haupt SH: The benefits of using humor in a management role. Surgical Services Management 1998 Jun; 4(6):45–47.

Kurtz S: Humor as a perioperative nursing management tool. Seminars in Perioperative Nursing 1999 Apr; 8(2):80–84.

Miller J: Humor—An empowerment tool for the 1990's. Empowerment in Organizations 1996; 4(2):16–21.

Morton RL, Kennedy MM: Advice from the experts. Experts address the professional concerns of healthcare executives. Healthcare Executive 1999 Mar/Apr; 14(2):44–45.

Preston P: Management strategies for encouraging creativity. Clinical Laboratory Management Review 1998 May/Jun; 12(3):185–192.

Saxton SE: What's funny about case management? Journal of Case Management 1997 Sum; 6(2):39–42.

Shearer R, Davidhizar R, Dowd SB: Humor: No materiel manager should be without it. Hospital Materiel Management Quarterly 1998 Aug; 20(1):29–36.

Summer C: On a wing and a prayer. Emergency Medical Services 1994 Apr; 23(4):16.

Pain and Pleasure

Bain L: The place of humour in chronic or terminal illness. Professional Nurse 1997 Jul; 12(10):713–715.

Dean RA: Humor and laughter in palliative care. Journal of Palliative Care 1997 Spr; 13(1):34–39.

Foltz-Gray D: Comic relief. Arthritis Today 1998 Nov; 12(6):26–30.

Kanninen M: Humor in palliative care: A review of the literature. International Journal of Palliative Nursing 1998 May/Jun; 4(3):110, 112–114.

McMullen LC: The correlation between humor and the chronic pain of arthritis. Journal of Holistic Nursing 1993 Mar; 11(1) 82–95.

Matz A, Brown ST: Humor and pain management: A review of current literature. Journal of Holistic Nursing 1998 Mar; 16(1): 71–88.

Nevo O, Keinan G, Teshimovsky-Arditi M: Humor and pain tolerance. Humor: International Journal of Humor Research 1993; 6(1):71–88.

Rhiner M, Dean GE, Ducharme S: Nonpharmacologic measures to reduce cancer pain in the home. Home Health Care Management & Practice 1996 Feb; 8(2):41–47.

Ward F: Using humor to deal with issues of loss and grief. Professional Medical Assistant 1992 Sep/Oct; 25(5):4.

Weisenberg M, Tepper I, Schwarzwald J: Humor as a cognitive technique for increasing pain tolerance. JMPT: Journal of Manipulative & Physiological Therapeutics 1997 Feb; 20(2):146.

Zillmann D, Rockwell S, Schweitzer K, Sundar SS: Does humor facilitate coping with physical discomfort? Motivation & Emotion 1993 Mar; 17(1):1–21.

Physiology of Laughter

Beaman N: Humor and health. Professional Medical Assistant Mar/Apr 1998; 31(2):24–25.

Boiten FA: The effects of emotional behaviour on components of the respiratory cycle. Biological Psychology 1998 Sep; 49(1–2): 29–51.

Docking K, Jordan FM, Murdoch BE: Interpretation and comprehension of linguistic humour by adolescents with head injury: A case-by-case analysis. Brain Injury 1999 Dec; 13(12): 953–972.

Fischman J: The brain's humor zone. U.S. News & World Report 1999 Apr 12; 126(14):49.

Fried I, Wilson CL, MacDonald KA, Behnke EJ: Electric current stimulates laughter. Nature 1998 Feb 12; 391(6668):650.

Koh KB: Emotion and immunity. Journal of Psychosomatic Research 1998 Aug; 45(2):107–115.

Lefcourt H, Davidson K, Prkachin K, Mills D: Humor as stress moderator in the prediction of blood pressure obtained during five stressful tasks. Journal of Research in Personality 1997 Dec; 31(4):523–542.

McCormack M: The laughter factor: It's more than a rumor—Humor is good for you. Volunteer Leader 1998 Spr; 39(1):9–10.

Mirsky S: Comic relief. Scientific American 1998 Apr; 278(4):22–23.

Nakajima A, Hirai H, Yoshino S: Reassessment of mirthful laughter in rheumatoid arthritis. Journal of Rheumatology 1999 Feb; 26(2):512–513.

Overeem S, Lammers GJ, van Dijk JG: Weak with laughter. Lancet 1999 Sep 4; 354(9181):838.

Peck G: Laughter: The internal pharmacy. Home Health Focus 1997 Sep; 4(4):25.

Perera S, Sabin E, Nelson P, Lowe D: Increases in salivary lysozyme and IgA concentrations and secretory rates independent of salivary flow rates following viewing of a humorous videotape. International Journal of Behavioral Medicine 1998; 5(2):118–128.

Ramachandran VS: The neurology and evolution of humor, laughter, and smiling: The false alarm theory. Medical Hypotheses 1998 Oct; 51(4):351–354.

Shammi P, Stuss DT: Humour appreciation: A role of the right frontal lobe. Brain 1999 Apr; 122(4): 657–666.

Psychological Aspects

Banning MR, Nelson DL: The effects of activity-elicited humor and group structure on group cohesion and affective responses. American Journal of Occupational Therapy 1987 Aug; 41(8):510–514.

Belanger HG, Kirkpatrick LA, Derks P: The effects of humor on verbal and imaginal problem solving. Humor: International Journal of Humor Research 1998; 11(1):21–31.

Barendsen K: Healing from depression: Prozac may get a lot of press, but many natural therapies help people find their way out of depression more safely. Yoga Journal 1996 Dec; 131:44, 48, 50, 52, 54–55, 140.

Buda B: Humor as therapeutic communication. The use of humor in psychotherapy. Dynamische Psychiatrie 1997; 30(5–6):305–319.

Burbach HJ, Babbitt CE: An exploration of the social functions of humor among college students in wheelchairs. Journal of Rehabilitation 1993 Jan/Feb/Mar; 59(1):6–9.

Burkhead EJ, Ebener DJ, Marini I: Humor, coping and adaptation to disability. Journal of Applied Rehabilitation Counseling 1996 Win; 27(4):50–53.

Carmi A: The role of humor in psychotherapy. Dynamische Psychiatrie 1997; 30(1–4):91–95.

Dossey L: Now you are fit to live; humor and health. Alternative Therapies in Health and Medicine 1996 Sep; 2(5):8–13, 98–100.

Galloway G: Psychological studies of the relationship of sense of humor to creativity and intelligence: A review. European Journal for High Ability 1994; 5(2):133–144.

Herzog TR: Gender differences in humor appreciation revisited. Humor: International Journal of Humor Research 1999; 12(4):411–423.

Martin RA, Kuiper NA: Daily occurrence of laughter: Relationships with age, gender, and Type A personality. Humor: International Journal of Humor Research 1999; 12(4):355–384.

Moran CC, Massam MM: Differential influences of coping humor and humor bias on mood. Behavioral Medicine 1999 Spr; 25(1):36–42.

Morreall J: The comic and tragic visions of life. Humor 1998; 11(4):333–355.

Perlini AH, Nenonen RG, Lind DL: Effects of humor on test anxiety and performance. Psychological Reports Jun 1999; 84(3 pt 2):1203–1203.

Ruch W, Carrell A: Trait cheerfulness and the sense of humour. Personality and Individual Differences 1998 Apr; 24(4):551–448.

Saunders PA: "You're out of your mind!": Humor as a face-saving strategy during neuropsychological examinations. Health Communication 1998; 10(4):357–372.

Thorson JA, Powell FC, Sarmany-Schuller I, Hampes WP: Psychological health and sense of humor. Journal of Clinical Psychology 1997 Oct; 53(6):605–609.

Westburg NG: Hope and humor: Using the Hope Scale in outcome studies. Psychological Reports 1999 Jun; 84(3 pt 1):1014–1020.

Wolfe DB: Boomer humor. American Demographics 1998 Jul; 20(7):22–23.

Special Patient Populations

A special kind of trust. Canadian Journal of Medical Technology 1988 Feb; 50(1):10–11.

Blood sampling that brings smiles! Canadian Journal of Medical Technology 1984 Dec; 46(4):232–233.

Adams P: Humor: Strong medicine. International Journal of Arts Medicine 1993 Sep; 2(2):22–23.

Arnold K: Cancer strikes the comic pages. Journal of the National Cancer Institute 1999 Mar 17; 91(6):499–500.

Bauer M: The use of humor in addressing the sexuality of elderly nursing home residents. Sexuality and Disability 1999 Sum; 17(2):147–156.

Buffum MD, Brod M: Humor and well-being in spouse caregivers of patients with Alzheimer's disease. Applied Nursing Research 1998 Feb; 11(1):12–18.

Clayton V: Send in the clowns. Nursing Times 1997 Aug 27; 93(35):36–37.

Cupples SA, Nolan MT, Augustine SM, Kynoch D: Perceived stressors and coping strategies among heart transplant candidates. Journal of Transplant Coordination 1998 Sep; 8(3):179–187.

Dowling JR: Laughter unlocks the memories of the heart: The radical role of humor in Alzheimer care. American Journal of Alzheimer's Disease 1997 Nov/Dec; 12(6):280–281.

Gillikin LS, Derks PL: Humor appreciation and mood in stroke patients. Cognitive Rehabilitation 1991 Sep/Oct; 9(5):30–35.

Grannis CJ: The ideal physical therapist as perceived by the elderly patient. Physical Therapy 1981 Apr; 61(4):479–486.

Hepler M: RCPs make Camp Superkids a big success. AARC Times 1991 Dec; 15(12): 22–23.

Houston DM, McKee KJ, Carroll L, Marsh H: Using humor to promote psychological wellbeing in residential homes for older people. Aging & Mental Health 1998 Nov; 2(4):328–332.

Kuiper NA, Martin RA, Olinger LJ, Kazarian SS, Jette JL: Sense of humor, self-concept, and psychological well-being in psychiatric inpatients. Humor 1998; 11(4):357–381.

Leibovitz A: Humor and dialysis. Edtna-Erca Journal 1998 Oct/Dec; 24(4):17–18.

Malone R: Look who's laughing. ASHA 1995 May; 37(5):96.

Marini I: The use of humour in counseling as a social skill for clients who are disabled. Journal of Applied Rehabilitation Counseling 1992 Fall; 23(3):30–36.

Nally AT: Nurse survivors face each new day with humor and hope. ONS News 1999 Jun; 14(6):1, 4–5.

Reeves PM, Merriam SB, Courtenay BC: Adaptation to HIV infection: The development of coping strategies over time. Qualitative Health Research 1999 May; 9(3):344–361.

Richman J: Jokes as a projective technique: The humor of psychiatric patients. American Journal of Psychotherapy 1996 Sum; 50(3):336–346.

Seltzer MM: Speculative gerontology revisited: The herd instinct. International Journal of Aging & Human Development 1992 Apr; 34(3):199–208.

Showalter SE, Skobel S: Hospice: Humor, heartache, and healing. American Journal of Hospice & Palliative Care 1996 Jul/Aug; 13(4):8–9.

Struthers J: An investigation into community psychiatric nurses' use of humour during client interactions. Journal of Advanced Nursing 1999 May; 29(5):1197–1204.

Witztum E, Briskin S, Lerner V: The use of humor with chronic schizophrenic patients. Journal of Contemporary Psychotherapy 1999 Fall; 29(3):223.

Young P: Why not laugh at old age? Elderly Care 1997 Aug/Sep; 9(4):46.

Stress Management

Tools for managing stress. Balanced Living 1996 Aug; 84:5–7.

Black JM: Writing your humor prescription: A stress management teaching strategy. Journal of Health Education 1999 Jul/Aug; 30(4):258–260.

Cann A, Holt K, Calhoun LG: The roles of humor and sense of humor in responses to stressors. Humor 1999; 12(2):177–193.

Gard CJ: Humor helps: Managing stress and anger. Current Health 1998 Apr/May; 24(8):22–23.

Hendrix BB: Stress for success. Medical Laboratory Observer 1993 Apr; 25(4):9.

Huston JL: Humor and stress: The workplace connection. Journal of the American Medical Record Association 1991 Apr; 62(4):47–49.

Jackson SH: The role of stress in anaesthetists' health and well-being. Acta Anaesthesiologica Scandinavica 1999 Jul; 43(6):583–602.

Kuhn PJ: Lecturing to the medical community and other difficult groups. Medical Laboratory Observer 1978 Jul; 19(7):83–86.

Kuiper NA, Martin RA: Laughter and stress in daily life: Relation to positive and negative affect. Motivation and Emotion 1998 Jun; 22(2):133–153.

More B: A laughing matter. Yoga Journal 1995 Aug; 123:28.

Palmer L: Did'ja hear the one about. . . Journal of AHIMA 1998 Sep; 69(8):21.

Perrin KM: Laugh at stress! Creative methods for teaching stress management. Journal of Health Education 1995 Sep/Oct; 26(5):309–310.

Perry PM: Stress busters. Materiels Management in Health Care 1999 Mar; 8(3):38–40.

Pitre S: The best medicine. Radiologic Technology 1996 Mar/Apr; 67(4):358.

Schwab P: Those who laugh . . . last! Professional Medical Assistant 1993 Mar/Apr; 26(2):8–10.

Umiker WO: Psycho-cybernetics: The proactive approach to stress management. MLO 1994 Nov; 26(11):28–30.

Therapeutic Humor

Bickley JB: Care for the caregiver: The art of self-care. Seminars in Perioperative Nursing 1998 Apr; 7(2):114–121.

Bjornson MR: They who laugh, last. Conscious Choice 1997 Jun; 10(3):46–47.

Brooks NA, Guthrie DW, Gaylord CG: Therapeutic humor in the family: An exploratory study. Humor: International Journal of Humor Research 1999; 12(2):151–160.

Galloway G, Cropley A: Benefits of humor for mental health: Empirical findings and directions for further research. Humor: International Journal of Humor Research 1999; 12(3):301–314.

Hammond P: Sick jokes. Health Service Journal 1997 Dec 18; 107(5584):30–31.

Hawk R: Spreading good cheer through laughter. AARC Times 1992 Feb; 16(2):19.

Hunter P: Humor therapy in home care. Caring 1997 Sep; 16(9):56–57.

Larkin M: How humour heals ills. Lancet 1998 Nov 7; 352(9139):1562.

Mycek S: Take two ginseng and call me in the morning. Trustee 1997 Jun; 51(6):14–16, 18–20.

Sharoff L, Kagan M: Tapestry of the mind-body spirit. Humor therapy: Laugh for the healing of it! Aspmn Pathways 1998 Spr; 7(1):12, 16.

Vergeer G, MacRae A: Therapeutic use of humor in occupational therapy. American Journal of Occupational Therapy 1993 Aug; 47(8):678–683.

Weir C: Living with IBD: A personal story. Canadian Association for Enterostomal Therapy 1994 Mar; 13(1):17–21.

Treating Patients

Gilston A: Humouring the patient. Anaesthesia 1999 Mar; 54(3):308.

Goldin E, Bordan T: The use of humor in counseling: The laughing cure. Journal of Counseling and Development 1999 Fal; 77(4):372–372.

McDonald M: Dr. Patch. U.S. News & World Report 1998 Dec 14: 125(23):56–59.

Madell SD: The decline and fall of bedside medicine. Journal of the American Academy of Physician Assistants 1991 Jul/Aug; 4(5):371–372.

Pector EA: Easy ways to make every patient feel special. Medical Economics 1998 Sep 21; 75(18):7–8.

Richard MA, Martin S, Gouvernet J, Folchetti G, Bonerandi JJ, Grob JJ: Humour and alarmism in melanoma prevention: A randomized controlled study of three types of information leaflet. British Journal of Dermatology 1999 May; 140(5): 909–914.

Rondberg TA: The real power of laughter. Chiropractic Journal 1998 Sep; 12(12):8, 16.

Santoro J: Send in the clown. Hospitals & Health Networks 1999 Apr; 73(4):14.

Setness PA: Lessons in humanity from corporate America and Patch Adams. Postgraduate Medicine 1999 Apr; 105(4):23.

Sponsler SB: The lesson Aloysius taught me. RN 1990 Jun; 53(6): 21–22.

Stanley D: Seeing the funny side of things can do more than just help you survive your job. Nursing Times 1999 Aug 25; 95(34):21.

Stone S: Good health through good humor. Nursing Homes 1999 Feb; 48(2):53–54.

Woodgate RL: Health professionals caring for chronically ill adolescents: Adolescents' perspectives. Journal of the Society of Pediatric Nurses 1998 Apr/Jun; 3(2):57–68.

Utilizing Humor in the Workplace

A spoonful of humor. Medical Laboratory Observer 1993 Dec; 25(12):50.

Leave 'em laughing. Emergency Medical Services 1992 Nov; 21(11):61.

Nurses clown around for health and nutrition. Homecare Education Management 1998 Nov; 3(11):174–176.

Bohl NK: Extinguishing burnout. Emergency 1996 Jul; 28(7):9.

Burchiel RN, King CA: Incorporating fun into the business of serious work: The use of humor in group processes. Seminars in Perioperative Nursing 1999 Apr; 8(2):60–70.

Davis A: Remember who you work for. Journal of the American Academy of Physician Assistants 1996 Jun; 9(6):15–16, 18.

Decker WH, Rotondo DM: Use of humor at work: predictors and implications. Psychological Reports 1999 Jun; 84(3):961–968.

Hartwell J: Injecting humor into healthcare. Nursing Focus 1997 Jul/Aug; 8–10, 16–17.

Jones JM: No silly symptoms. Physician Assistant 1989 Aug; 13(8):136.

Kesler L: Learning the value of an "F": A message to new graduates. Advance for Physical Therapists & PT Assistants 1998 Jun 1; 9(22):35–37.

Leo J: Chortle while you work. U.S. News & World Report 1999 Apr 26:19.

McGhee P: Rx: Laughter. RN 1998 Jul; 61(7):50–53.

Makin R: Laugh? I nearly re-joined the NHS. Nursing Times 1999 Mar 24; 95(12):22.

Malloy J: And now for something completely different . . . using humor effectively in the workplace. Intech 1999 Oct; 46(10): 75–76.

Murphy JF: Putting a chuckle in therapy. Advance for Physical Therapists 1998 Apr 6; 9(14):50.

Payne D, Raper M: The last laugh. Nursing Times 1999 Dec 29; 95(5):24–25.

Porter-O'Grady T: Laughter lightens our load. Nursing Management 1999 Sep; 30(9):4.

Siddall L: Transporting in style. Emergency 1995 Jun; 27(6):70.

Stevens L: Take my patient, please: Medical humor on the net. Medicine on the Net 1998 Jul; 4(6):7–10.

Weaver ST, Wilson CN: Addiction counselors can benefit from appropriate humor in the work setting. Journal of Employment Counseling 1997 Sep; 34(3):108–114.

Whaley C: Humor: Prescription for the work place. Journal of Diagnostic Medical Sonography 1993 Mar/Apr; 9(2):88–89.

White AA: Compassionate patient care and personal survival in orthopaedics. A 35-year perspective. Clinical Orthopaedics & Related Research 1999 Apr; 361:250–260.

AUTHOR INDEX

Akin, Renea, p. 161
Barry, Dave, p. 185
Bennett, Doug(2), p. 21, p. 26
Bennett, Howard J. (2), p. 61, p. 145
Bentley, Stuart A., p. 17
Birtcher, Cecil, p. 138
Black, Jan (2), p. 152, p. 153
Brone, Jeff, p. 51
Bruhn, John G., p. 125
Burnette, Norman L., p. 133
Cardinale, Valentine, p. 63
Carlson, Bruce, p. 101
Carlstedt, Bruce C., p. 78
Chase, Linda M., p. 150
Chesney, Alan P., p. 125
Dandy, Dan, p. 30
Daniel, Erno S., p. 147
Demers, Bob, p. 182
Devermann, Arthur W., p. 69
Dickinson, Ben, p. 178
DiMaggio, Charles, p. 135
Dirckx, John H., p. 151
Dolan, John, p. 154
Drazic, Sheila, p. 165
Dunea, George, p. 144
Fraser, F. Clarke, p. 140
Friedman, Bruce A., 109
Geetter, Joan, p. 117
Goldwyn, Robert M. (3), p. 75, p. 89, p. 123
Gordon, Leo A., p. 87
Grayson, Mary (3), p. 82, p. 90, p. 184
Hall, Sharon P., p. 52
Hanavan, Francis V., p. 146
Hansten, Philip D., p. 183
Hasegawa, Elizabeth A. J., p. 93
Helmholz, H. F., Jr., p. 131
Herman, Joseph, p. 7
Hoare, Tricia, p. 136
Hunt, Dexter (2), p. 159, p. 173
Ince, Victor, p. 98
Jenkins, Mary, p. 169
Johnson, Pam, p. 50
Keats, Theodore E., p. 180

Kirschbaum, Joel, p. 94
Kovacek, Peter, p. 29
Labelle, Art, p. 139
Lally, James F., p. 79
Laster, Leonard, p. 107
Leahy, Maribeth, p. 164
Levy, Gabor B., p. 10
Lucia, Jeff, p. 25
McBrayer, Jeff, p. 67
McNab, Warren, p. 62
Malone, Russell L. (2), p. 19, p. 177
Mason, Allen, p. 134
Matkin, Ralph E., p. 154
Merton, Daniel, p. 34
Moran, Jeffrey B., p. 148
Morin, Karen H., p. 99
Morris, Barbara M., p. 33
Mueller, Bruce A., p. 78
Neely, Elaine, p. 53
Nelson, Greg, p. 167
Nephew, Kathy, p. 164
Novatnack, Ellen, p. 57
Nowak, Steve, p. 115
O'Connor, Thomas W. (2), p. 113, p. 163
O'Malley, Kevin Shea, p. 13
O'Rourke, Eileen (2), p. 53, p. 57
Ott, Bill, p. 66
Parry, Anne, p. 127
Paskevitch, Yuska-Marie, p. 102
Penn, Barbara, p. 77
Pentecost, William R., 85
Plagakis, Jim, p. 40
Pruchnicki, Alec, p. 73
Quinn, Campion, p. 41
Quinn-O'Connor, Robert, p. 53
Radcliffe, Mark, p. 100
Ramsey, Michael Kirby (2), p.114, p. 166
Rothstein, Jules M. (3), p. 9, p. 95, p. 105
Savinese, Stanley J., p. 80
Schweon, Steven J. (2), p. 53, p. 57
Shaffer, Michael J., p. 128
Shaughnessy, Allen F., p. 149
Sitzman, Kathy, p. 32

Smith, Brendan, p. 171
Somers, Martha, p. 56
Sorbello, Joseph G., 155
Sredl, Darlene, p. 121
Stenger, Amber, p. 49
Tapson, Victor F., p. 65
Tate, Colleen Wedderburn, p. 170
Teagarden, J. Russell, p. 3
Thomas, Cliff, p. 55
Thompson, Edward M., p. 149
Tiger, Steven (2), p. 15 p. 46
Trout, Susan (2), p. 53, p. 57

VanSant, Ann F., p. 179
Vickers, Montgomery, p. 27
Vietenthal, Pat, p. 181
vön Koln Kleinmüntz, B., p. 64
Wagner, Lynn, p. 86
Warn, March L. (2), p. 39, p. 47
Whitman, Neal A., p. 11
Wijesinha, Sanjiva, p. 119
Wolfe, Jeannette, p. 45
Wolman, David (5), p. 5, p. 35, p. 83, p. 103, p. 143
Woltersdorf, Mitchel A., p. 132
Yeager, J. W., p. 187